SHiBARi

from Basic to Suspension

Published by Tabou Ediitons, an imprint of Editions de l'Eveil, France
www.tabou-editions.com

Tabou Edition is a registrated trademark of Editions de l'Eveil.

1.2500.BP.05/21

Printed in China by Book Partners China Ltd.
Cover and Interior design by Terry Marx
First Edition

Paper Edition : ISBN 978-2-36326-092-5
Digital pdf Edition – ISBN 978-2-36326-734-4
Digital ePub Edition – ISBN 978-2-36326-735-1
Édition papier en français – ISBN 978-2-36326-091-8
Édition numérique pdf en français – ISBN 978-2-36326-732-0
Édition numérique ePub en français – ISBN 978-2-36326-733-7

PHILIPPE BOXIS

SHiBARi

from Basic to Suspension

A pocket guide
20 lessons
step-by-step illustrations

Tabou

Contents

Floor positions — 56

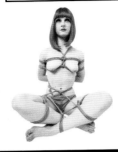

Sitting cross-legged • #4
58

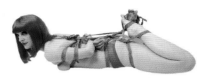

Hogtie • #5 — **70**

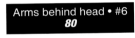

Arms behind head • #6
80

Finishing work on
the legs • #8
96

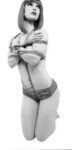

Floor improvisation • #9
106

Hands crossed
on chest • #7
88

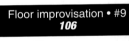

Sitting with eyes and
mouth bound • #12
130

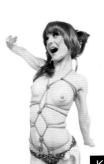

Karada on the arm • #11
124

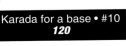

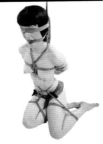

Karada for a base • #10
120

Contents

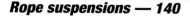

Rope suspensions — 140

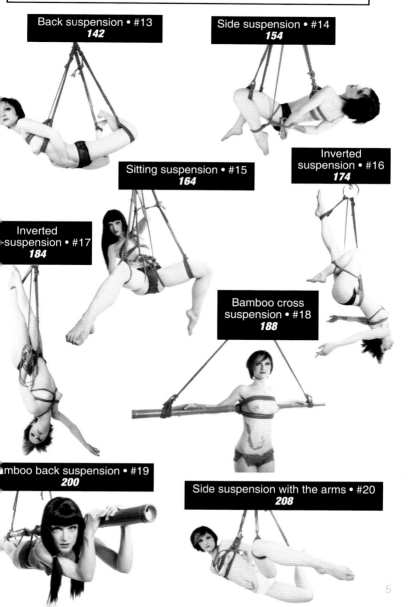

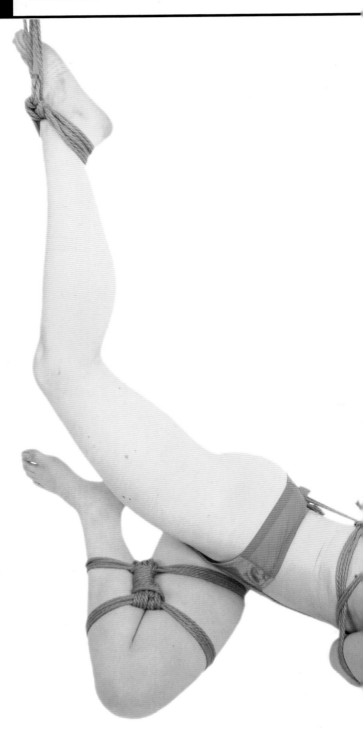

Disclaimer

Neither the author nor the publisher can accept any responsibility for any harm or damage whatsoever resulting from the application of the ideas or exercises described in this book. The reader must be fully aware that any inaccurate practice of the positions described below and of Shibari in general, including omissions or inconsistency, not in accordance with the instructions given in the present book, might cause injury. Likewise, the author and publisher cannot take any responsibility for traumas that might be caused by the use of ropes and Shibari equipment in general.

Shibari, sex and any BDSM-related practice are for consenting adults. The application of Shibari techniques and BDSM practices, as well as the use of sex toys, may be dangerous if the necessary precautions and care have not been strictly observed. Before you attempt any Shibari activity, read all of the instructions in this book and make sure you respect all the safety measures required for your activities to proceed in 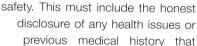 safety. This must include the honest disclosure of any health issues or previous medical history that might keep you or your partners from practising Shibari in complete safety.

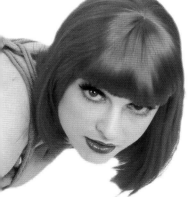

You should know, finally, that the use of drugs and alcohol can affect your judgment seriously and thus increase any risks.

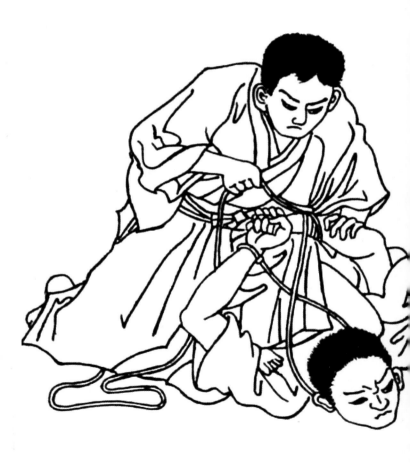

The origins of shibari

Shibari is a Japanese erotic speciality that consists of binding the human form with art and refinement.

The practice of Shibari is ancient. It began many centuries ago as a warrior technique in which prisoners were bound and restrained in a ritual way.
Each crime had its own specific binding technique that also took the prisoner's social position into account.

During the Tokugawa period (15th and 16th centuries), the Penal Code provided for four kinds of punishment. Among them was rope suspension, which was considered the most serious punishment, because it could lead to death.

During the Edo period (1603-1869), *Hojōjutsu* – literally, "the art of rope binding" – was considered to be a martial art, whose rules were:

• Never enable the prisoner to wriggle out of his ties.
• Never cause physical or mental aftereffects.
• Never disclose the techniques in use.
• Make sure that the result is pleasant-looking.

It is the last rule that cultivated the emergence of what we know today as Shibari.

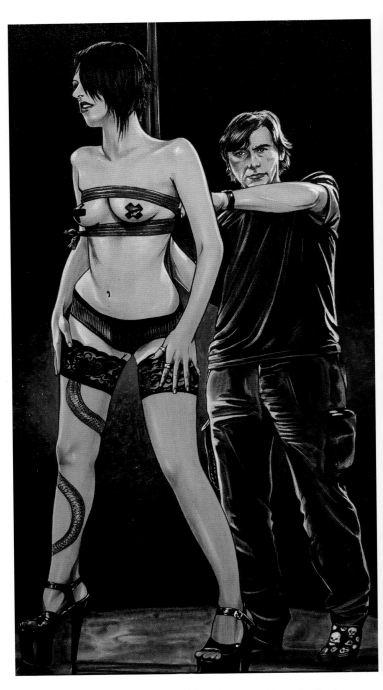

Philippe Boxis as seen by David Ducarteron (www.david.ducarteron.blogspirit.com)

Ask Philippe Boxis...

…how he came to practise Shibari… He'll answer that he has always loved tying up his girlfriends, and ropes have always been part of his everyday life!

As a result, Philippe Boxis is a self-taught man. Ropes are omnipresent in his life. For him, the beauty and vulnerability of a tied-up woman evokes the strongest fantasies.

Inspired by Japanese bondage iconography, he made a decision at the age of fifty to go to Japan to find the masters of his life's art. When he met Steve Osada, it was an absolute revelation: he could finally put a name to what he had always been feeling deep within himself.

That's how Philippe, a professional photographer, started a new life. From then on, he combined photography with Shibari… or rather, he put photography to good use for his art in order to share it with the world.

Shibari, an art of living

Philippe's approach is aesthetic above all: a work performed in concert with the body. In his ropes, a woman becomes a piece of sculpture; she is enhanced, made gorgeous.

His work is quick, neat, unadorned and avoids excess. He adapts to the physical characteristics of each of his models: his work might adapt to a suppleness, a morphology, a model's hair, a clothing style, or something else.

He draws his inspiration from his environment, and incorporates the elements: he might find inspiration from a nearby wall, a tree, a rock, an armchair, a chest of drawers, a table, or an inspiring object.

His strong point is improvisation. He likes listening to his imagination.

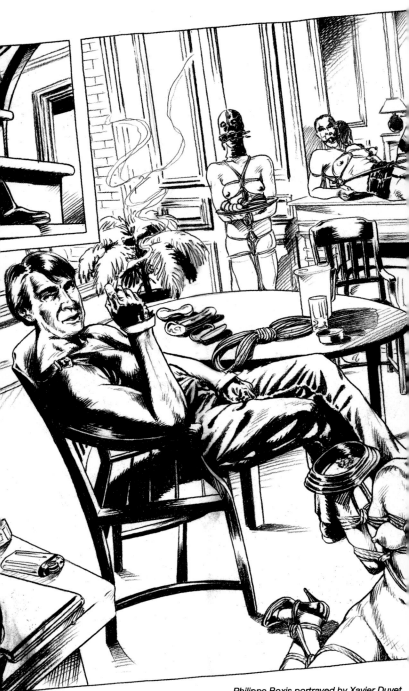

Philippe Boxis portrayed by Xavier Duvet
(www.xavierduvet.com), from the book « Les maîtresses - Leçons de prédatrices » (Tabou Éditions, 2011)

His goal: sharing

Philippe helps democratize Shibari with his workshops, performances, and public shows in France and around the world. He has shared his art in locations that include Boundcon (Munich), Nuit Démonia (Paris), Clinic Party (Amsterdam), Torture Garden (London), Japan Shibari Tour (Tokyo, Osaka, Nagoya, Kobe), SM Club (Rome), and many more.
In the same vein, he contributed to the series *"Paris Enquêtes Criminelles"* on TF1, *"Xanadu"* on ARTE, and he took part in the animated short film *"La Femme à Cordes"* by Vladimir Mavounia-Kouka.

Philippe Decoufle asked him to integrate ropes into the dance performance he directed, *"Cœurs Croisés"*, which was presented in the Palais-Royal gardens (Paris).

Finally, Philippe Boxis's DVD, *"Leçons de cordes"*, was met with great success.

A meeting with the audience

When Philippe Boxis uncoils the first of his ropes, the model has already begun to surrender to his creativity, with her senses awakening. The smell, the sound of the rope as it slips around her body, the feeling of rope over her skin, these sensations thrill her to the utmost. His fingers flutter around, the gestures soft – but the intention is firm. There seems to be nothing else around the couple; everyone in the audience holds his breath… Nothing but this nude, gorgeous woman – and this man who transforms her into a goddess. Philippe's girlfriend and model Miia tells us:

"I admire his professionalism and his kind-hearted nature. I always feel respected and secure with him. Philippe possesses the rare skill of sensing women intuitively.
The freshness of his inspiration, delicate eroticism, both sensuous and torrid, absolute love of the weaker sex, harmonious and inspired adaptation of Shibari to the Western culture… These are just a few of the sensations that come to my mind as I admire the result of his work. A work that is continually developing, and that brings new sensations at every session."

Welcome, reader: it's time to discover this world.

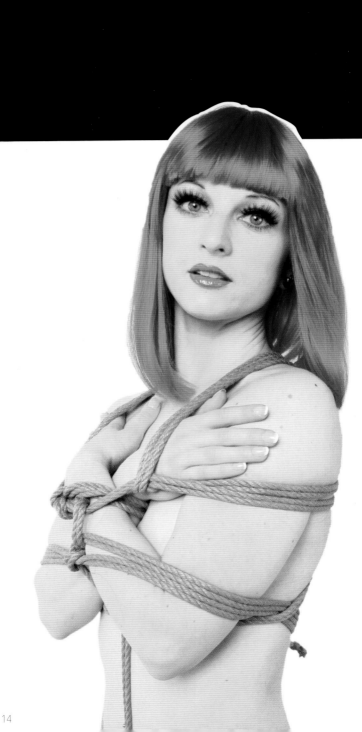

Basic knowledge

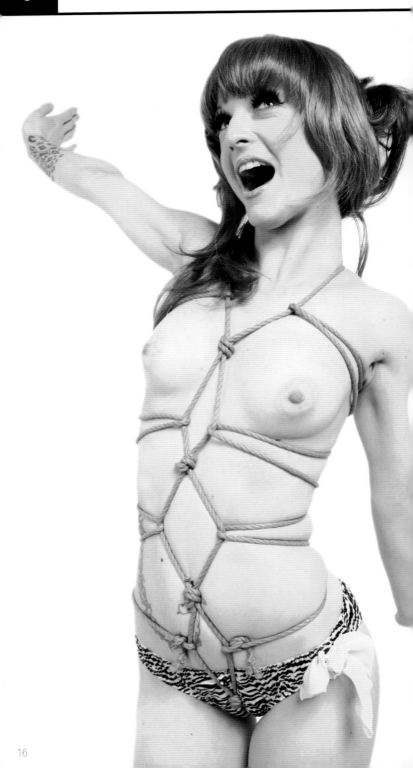

Safety, rules and advice

- Regularly ask about and check on the model's well-being.
- Always be ready to listen to the model, and never leave her unattended.
- Never forget that the rigger is the person responsible, and consequently he or she will have to take the initiative in untying if necessary, sometimes against the model's opinion.
- Ensure that when you pull on a rope you never do it too quickly, especially if the rope is in contact with the skin, and always create a protection with your fingers for rope that has contact with the most delicate parts of the body.
- In order not to tangle the ropes, it's important to untie them systematically in the reverse order from the binding process. It's even more important that you follow this rule when undoing a suspension.
- Never untie the chest before the model can touch the floor with either both hands, or both feet.
- Untie the model immediately if for any reason she feels unwell.
- In any situation, you must never panic.
- It's often wiser to untie the ropes calmly in order to reassure the model.
- In case of emergency, necessity, or if a knot becomes jammed, use EMT scissors or round-tip scissors to cut the ropes (and keep in mind that you must never untie the chest before the model could lean on the floor with both hands or both feet).
- Strength isn't necessarily required to lift a bound person. Once the ties are made around the upper body and the first leg, you only have to pull the second leg up. For the model, the suspension only begins when she leaves the ground completely.
- A suspension will always be a physical performance for the model; thus it must be carried out over a short length of time..

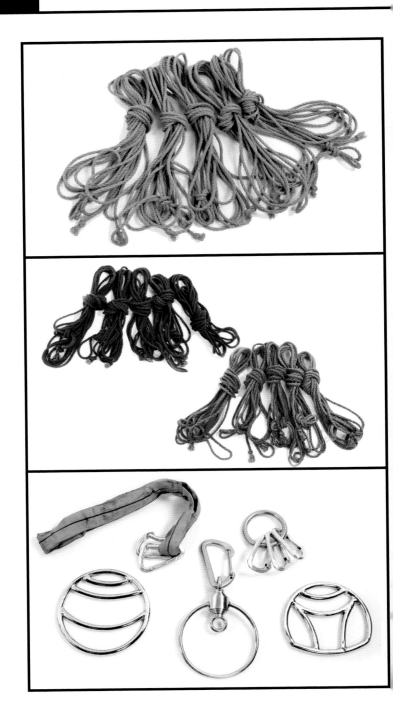

Equipment

For a good start, you only need a set of five 25-30ft pieces of rope. That will be enough for you to learn the basics and work on the floor. The ropes must be jute or hemp, ecru or dyed, preferably 4 or 5mm (1/6" or 1/5") for working on the floor.

Once you have acquired the basics, the ideal setup consists of six 25-30ft pieces of rope, 6mm thick: you can do everything with this set, including suspensions. For the latter, a secure suspension point is essential. When you're ready for suspensions, add to your equipment a specific ring that enables you to separate each rope properly; you can also use rock-climbing carabiners. A lifting sling and a pair of safety scissors will complete your equipment.

Before you learn a particular rope-folding method, you need to understand why it's important. When you practise Shibari, you must always work in continuity, with your ropes folded in half. This means you always start from the middle, and the junction with the next rope is done upon the ends of the first one. From this, it's obvious that if you want to have the two ends on the same level when finishing your work, you need to start precisely from the middle. There are several rope-folding methods; it doesn't matter which one you choose to use as long as your method allows you to locate the middle easily.

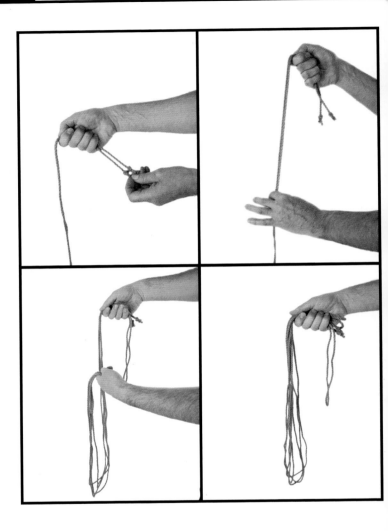

Place the two ends of the rope side by side and hold them tight in your right hand to prevent the ropes from slipping.

Slide your other hand along the rope to grab the end, but maintain the tension on the two parts to keep an equal length.

Once you find the middle, pinch it with your left thumb and index finger, still holding the two ends in your right hand.

Fold the rope in half as you place the middle about 8 inches from the two ends. Then fold the rope in half again, level with the ends to keep the middle apart.

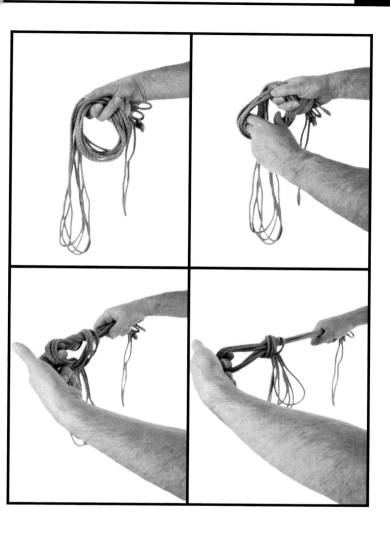

Form a rounded loop by using the palm of your hand. The loop must be held by the same hand but be sure to hold it lightly so you can loosen it gradually when you tighten the knot. Reach your left hand into the loop and grab the ropes. Pull them back through the loop. Just pull on the two parts enough to find a good balance between having enough tension to keep the knot tight, and avoiding the possibility of the knot untying easily.

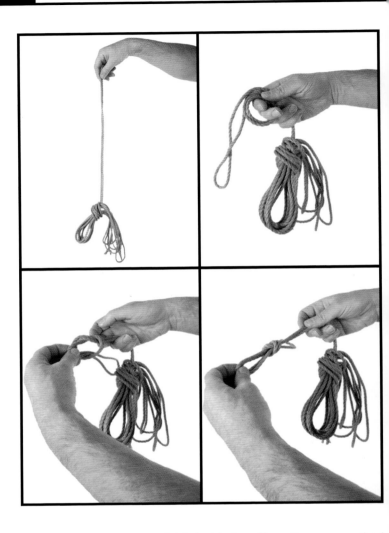

With the middle now completely isolated, we'll use the same method with the remaining part. This is so you can find the middle of the rope immediately once you've untied it.

Form a loop in the same way, wide enough to reach two fingers into it, grab the rope and pull it back through the loop. Tighten the knot by pulling on the two ends.

Your rope is now ready to go into action – you should know that the starting point will always be the middle of the rope you've just located.

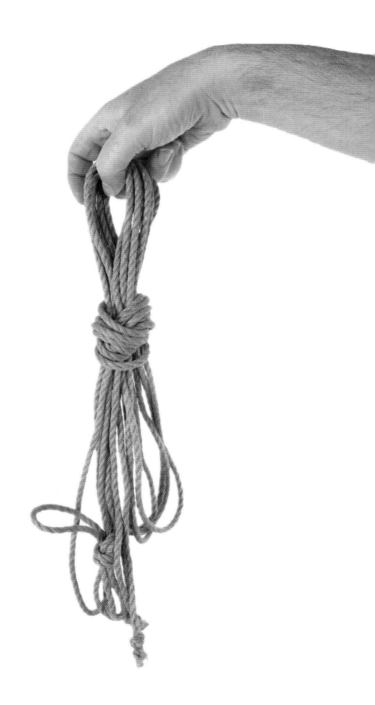

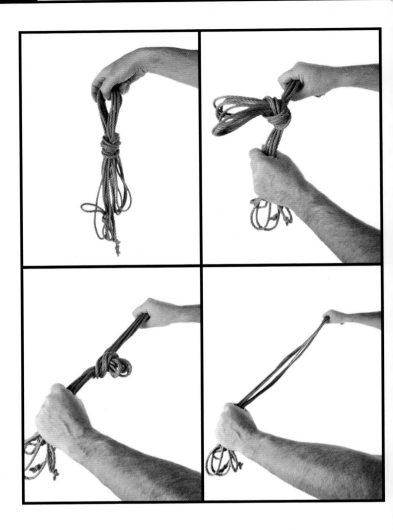

Untie the rope with both hands so you can separate the two parts properly. Give it a pull to untie the loop.

You'll have to teach yourself to fold and untie the ropes quickly; it will determine the good start of your Shibari as well as the continuity of your work during your binding. Now that the rope is partly untied, you just have to do the same for the middle.

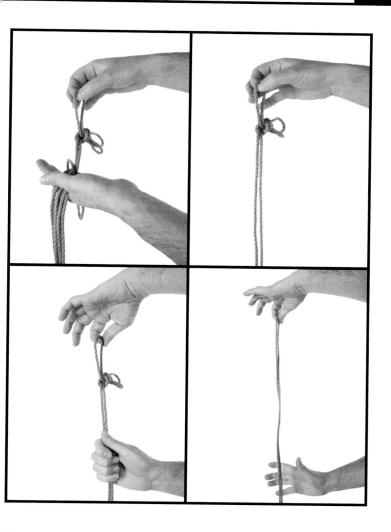

Be sure to keep the part containing the middle in your hand. Pinch the middle with two fingers so you won't lose it. Pull on the two ends to untie the loop.

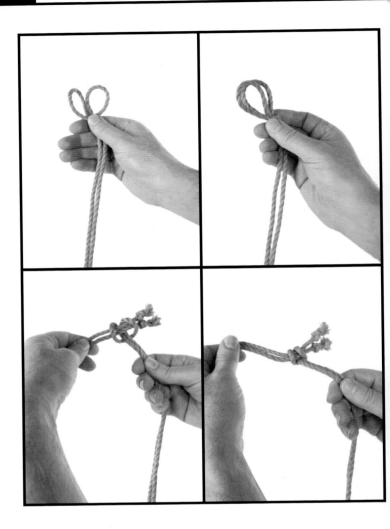

Fold the new rope in half from the middle in order to form a lark's head. Tuck the ends of the previous rope through the bight. Tighten the knot. If the middle has been respected, the two rope ends should be on the same level.

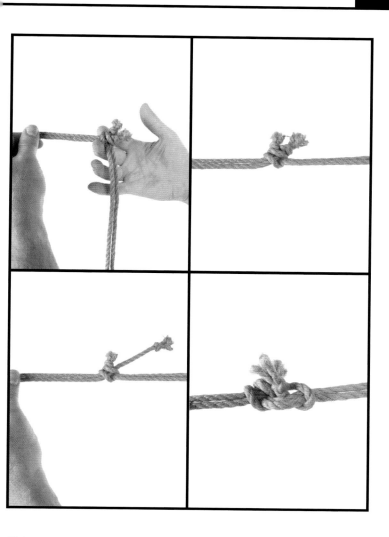

Slide the lark's head to the end of the rope. The tension on the two ropes will make it a self-locking system. On the contrary, if you give the junction some slack, it'll allow you to untie it if necessary. In case the two ends are not aligned, you can solve this by tying an overhand knot with the little bit that's poking out. That will make it more aesthetically pleasing, and allows you to maintain an equal tension on each of the two lengths. **Be careful:** depending on each model's morphology, you won't always do the junction with the next rope in the same place.

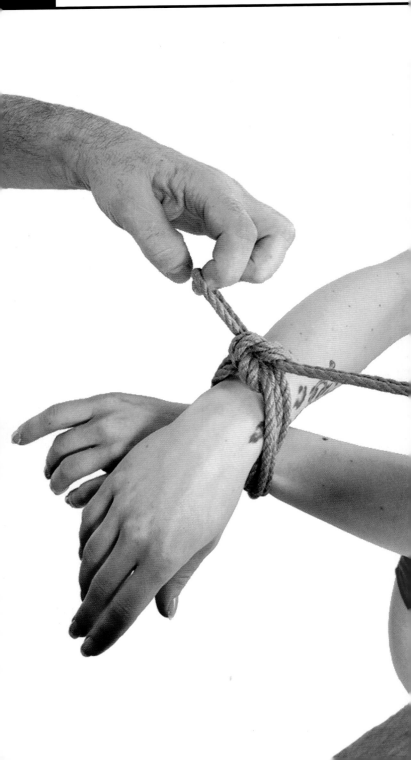

Basic ties: Hands

The basic tie is what you'll use for tying the model's hands without cutting off the blood circulation, and you'll also use this method on different parts of the body.

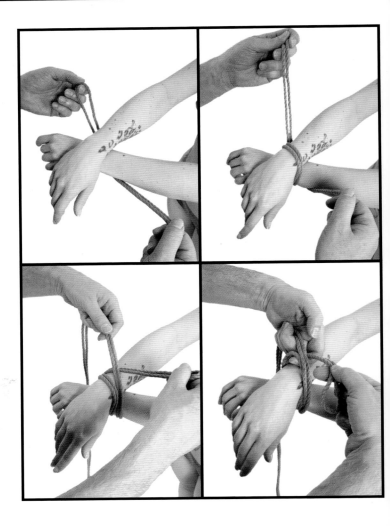

Start by wrapping the rope twice around the wrists while keeping the two winding coils parallel to one another. Make sure you keep a two-finger space between the model's wrists, and the ropes.

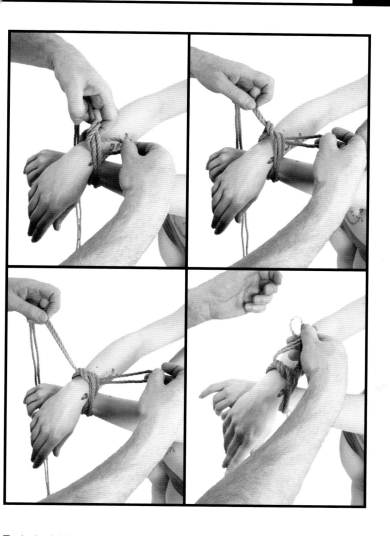

Tuck the bight underneath so you can take the whole wrap. Tighten it lightly, then start tying a square knot, while making sure there is a free space left.

The remaining bight is the one you'll use later, either taking it to impose a particular restraint in a certain position, or you can use it to secure a suspension.

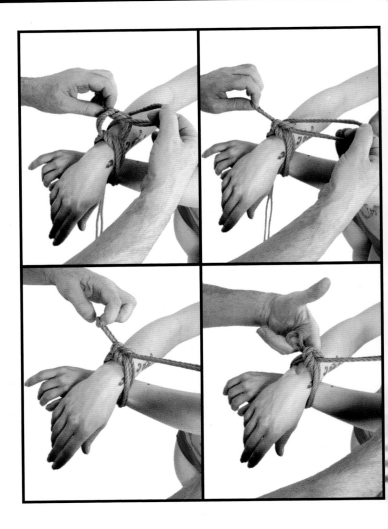

Finish the square knot and check that you have left a two-finger space between the ropes and the wrists.

Basic ties: Legs

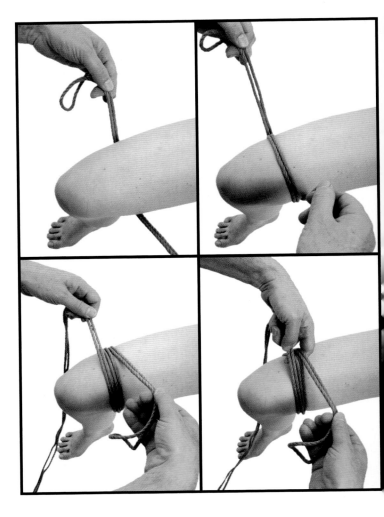

Apply the same method above the knee. The bight will come in handy afterwards.

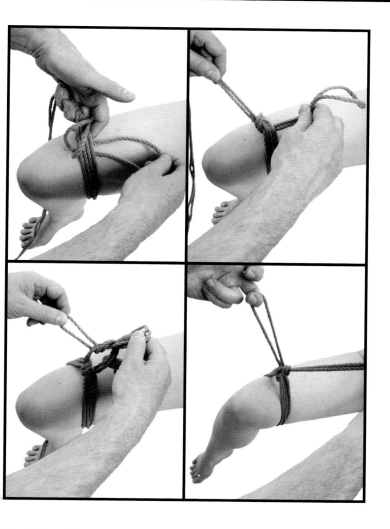

Check to make sure you have a two-finger space between the ropes and the leg.

This tie will be useful for suspensions.

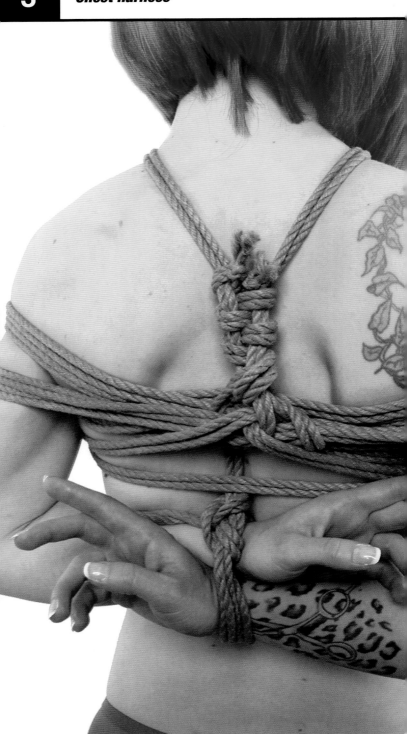

Chest harness

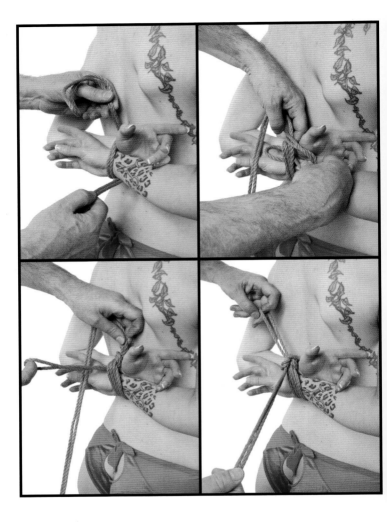

Now we'll apply what we just learned, but this time with the wrists behind the back.

Wrap the rope around the wrists twice.

Use the whole wrap to tie a square knot.

Leave the bight long: this will allow you to adjust the space between the rope and the wrists when you tighten. You'll be able

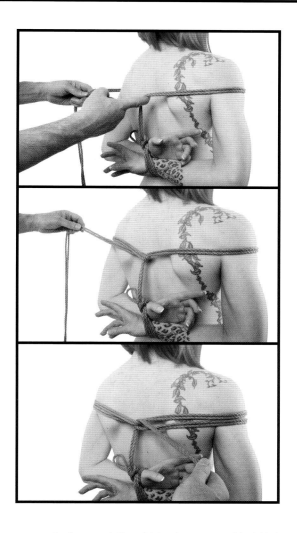

Pull the rope up to the model's mid-back area, and hold it here while you wrap it above the breasts a first time. Create a counter-tension in the mid-back where you're holding the rope. Wrap the rope the other way around a second time, above the breasts, and then adjust the counter-tension.

Holding the rope in the middle will allow you to work in symmetry. This tension and counter-tension system is the very principle of Shibari, and it's very important to apply it naturally. It will allow you, during your improvisational work, to tighten ropes that would have been left "slack" or "hanging loose".

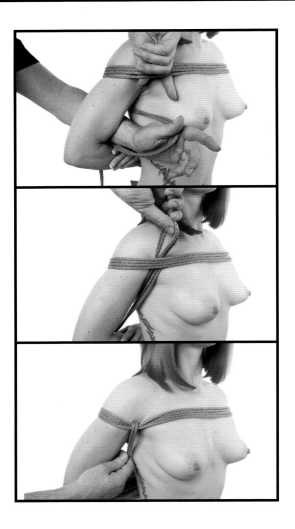

Always make sure your winds are flat and parallel to each other. Next, we'll secure the ropes so they can't slide up.

From top to bottom, reach two of your fingers under the wrap to grab the rope; tuck the bight slowly up and under the wrap, while being careful not to pinch the model's skin.

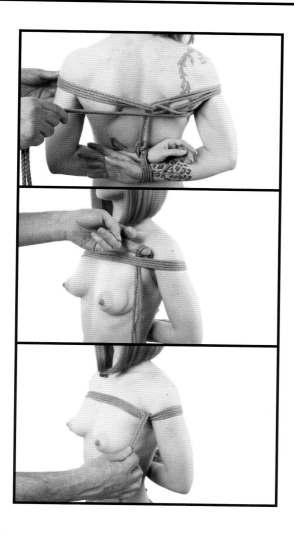

Bring the rope across the back and do the same on the other side.
This increases tightening, which is why you need to find the right balance
in the tension

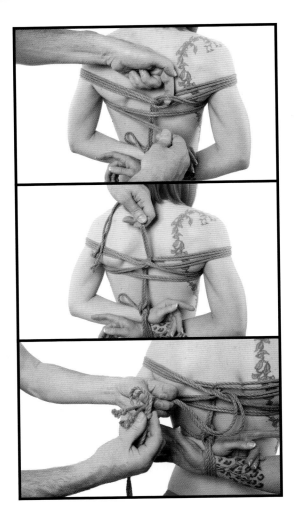

Return to the mid-back area and adjust the counter-tension. Prepare the loop on the next rope to work in continuity.

Pay attention to the place where you adjust the counter-tension: it must not be on an isolated rope, but in a loop where tension is already applied.

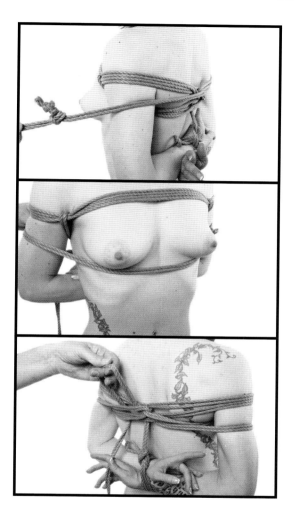

Now we'll wrap the rope twice below her breasts the same way.

Begin by wrapping the rope below the breast; adjust the counter-tension, then wrap the rope a second time in the opposite direction.

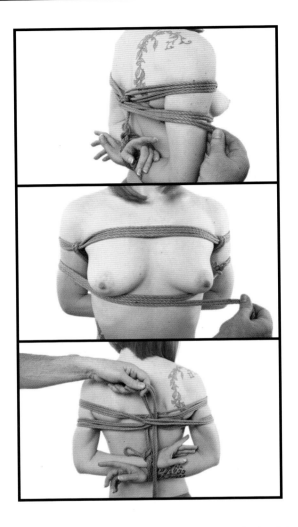

Keep the ropes parallel to each other, then return to the back to finish.

Now we're going to tie a first stopper knot (or overhand knot).

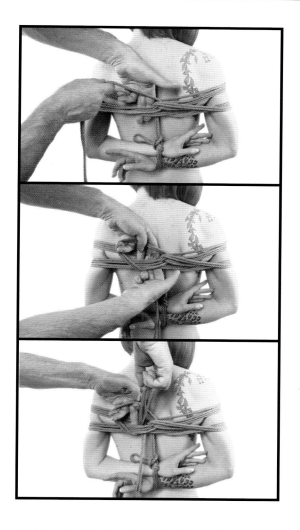

While maintaining the tension, form the loop of the overhand knot.

Pull the rope through the loop with your other hand.

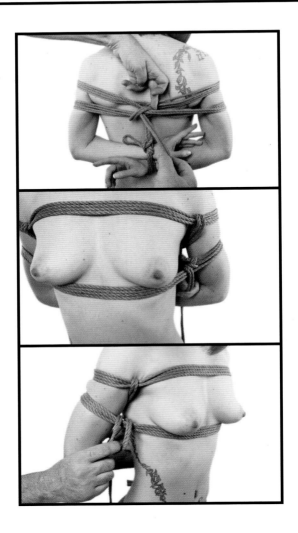

Tighten the knot.

Secure it between the chest and arms as you've done before, but this time below the breasts.

Do the same on the other side.

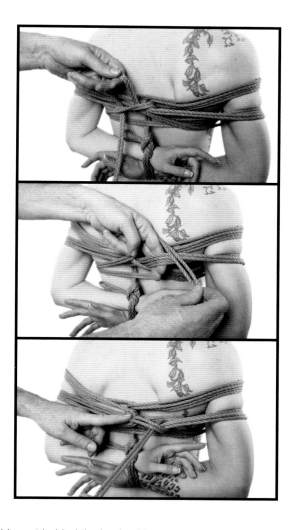

Finish this part behind the back with a second overhand knot.

The first knot was not essential, but it's useful to separate the different parts.

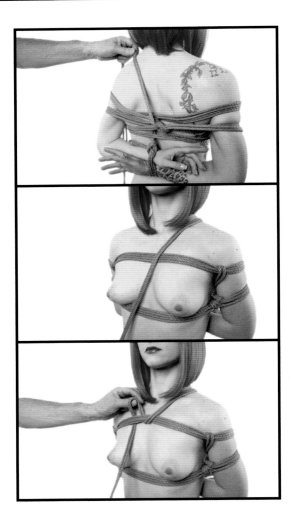

Bring the rope up to the shoulder.

Tuck the rope underneath the upper wrap on the chest.

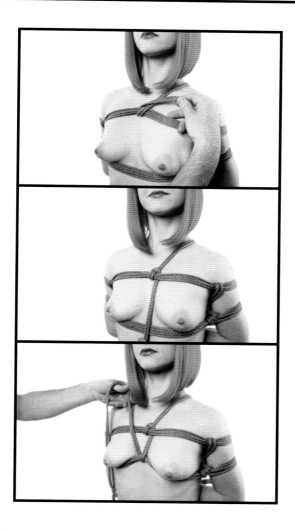

Bring the rope over the first shoulder strap, then once more under the upper wrap on the chest. The little coil of rope that you just created allows you to create a tension point without tying a knot. This is for aesthetics, but it's also useful if you need to reduce any slack in the ropes. We'll call it a "tension loop" from now on. Take the lower wrap on the chest and apply a light tension.

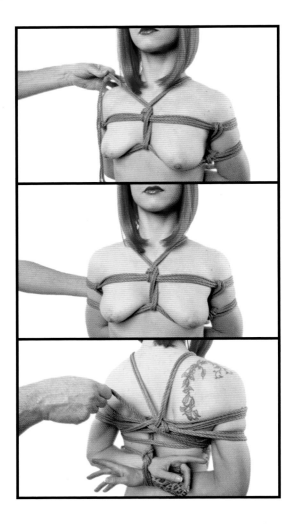

Tuck the rope under the first shoulder strap, in the direction that will allow you to create an opposite tension, as well as the second shoulder strap. Finish the piece behind the back.

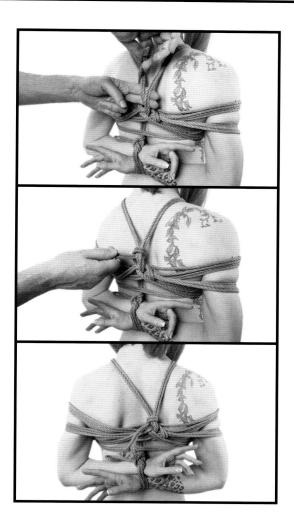

Tie the last overhand knot.

We are going to study a few possible variants.

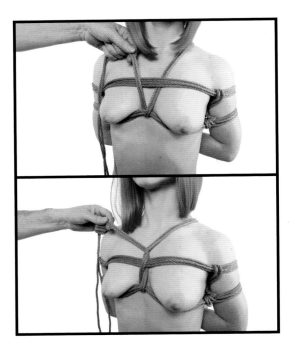

Tuck the shoulder rope straight under the upper wrap on the chest and take the lower wrap. Apply opposite tension by using the shoulder rope to create a second shoulder strap.

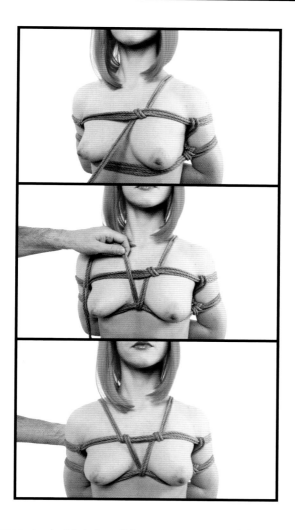

Another way to do this is to coil the rope once around the upper wrap. Take the lower wrap and coil the rope once more around the upper wrap. Create the second shoulder strap and finish the piece behind the back.

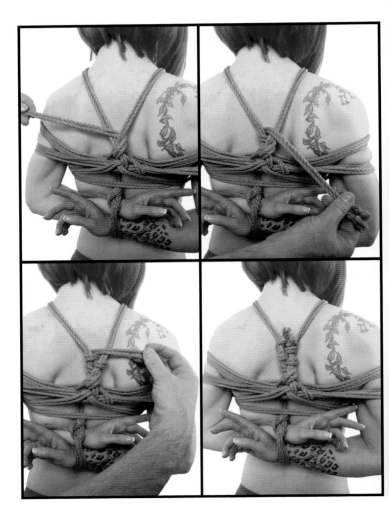

However, to have a clean finish means you'll need to get rid of this excess rope elegantly.

One solution is to wind it all the way up the shoulder straps, one time underneath, one time over. No extra knot is needed.

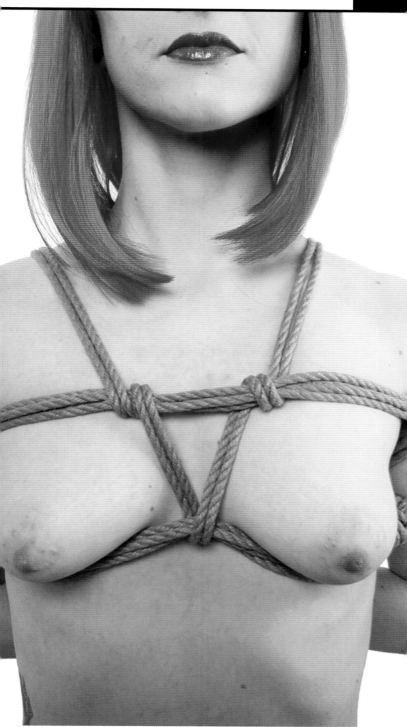

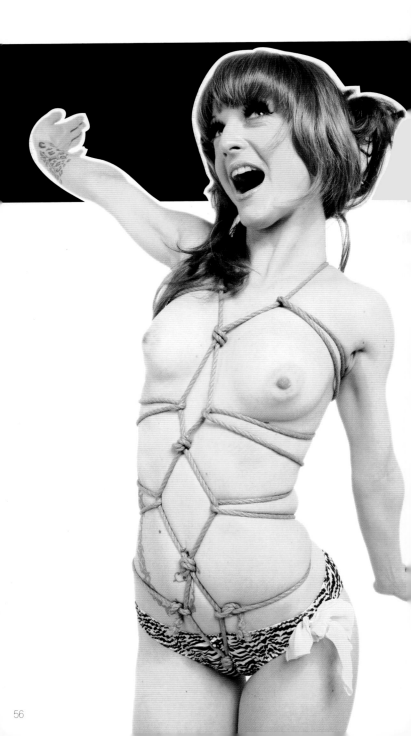

Floor

Positions

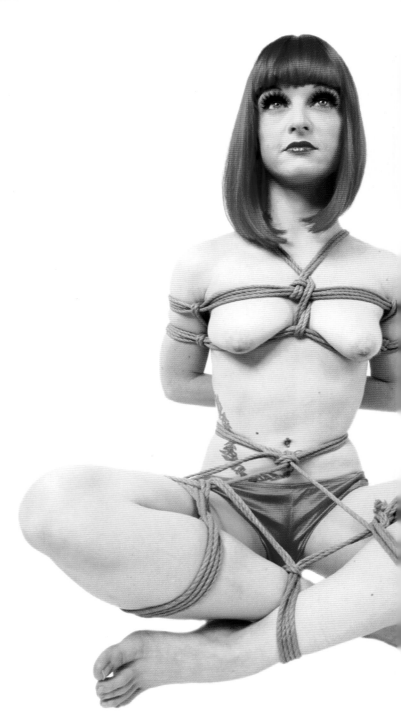

Sitting cross-legged

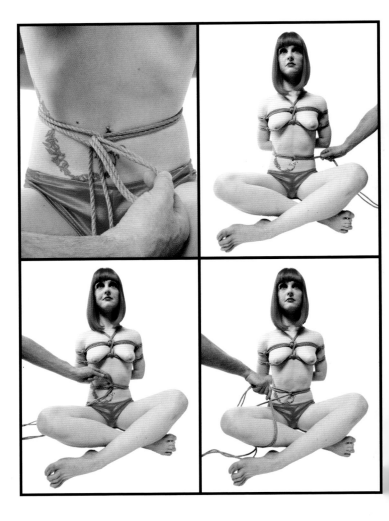

From the "Chest harness with arms bound" (lesson #3), we'll start from the waist and bring the work down to the legs. (You can also do it in continuity by adding a rope behind the back.)

Start with a lark's head at the model's mid-waist area.

Wrap the rope a second time in counter-tension the other way around. Take the wrap in mid-waist again, then bring the rope down to her leg.

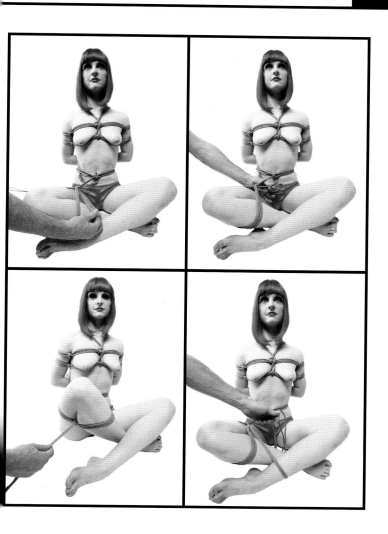

Wrap the rope a first time around the leg as you position the tension point in the middle of the fold. Wrap the rope a second time, adjust the tension on the same point, and secure it under the knee using the rope running along the outside. Bring the rope back to the tension point on the inside, and you can start to tie both ankles.

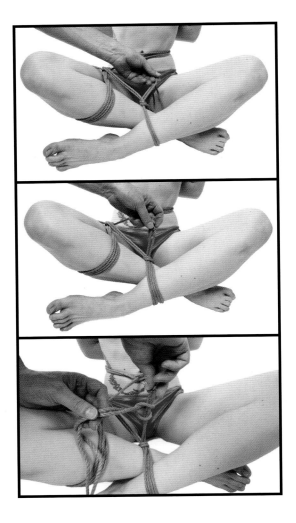

Wrap the rope once, adjust the counter-tension, then wrap the rope a second time.
Move on to the next rope using the same technique.
Bring the rope to the other leg and repeat the work in symmetry.

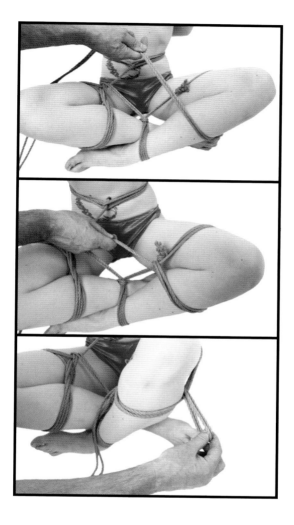

Take the folded leg and create the tension point over the fold, just as you did on the first leg.

Wrap the rope twice.

Tuck the rope under the knee to create symmetry, and use the outside ropes as anchor points again.

Bring the rope back to the inside and adjust the tension point.

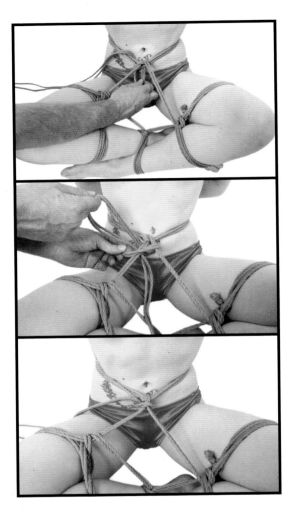

Bring the rope back to the central point at the model's mid-waist area.
Tie an overhand knot while maintaining the tension and cinch it.

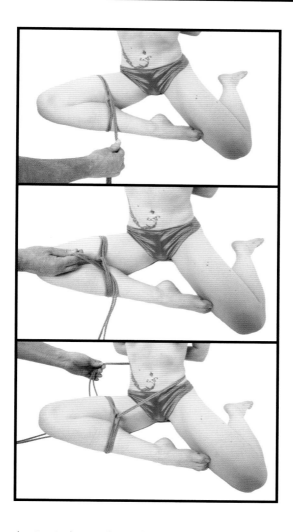

We are going to study **a variant with legs aside.**
Start with a lark's head in the middle of the folded leg.
Wrap the rope twice using the tension and counter-tension technique,
then bring the rope up to the waist.

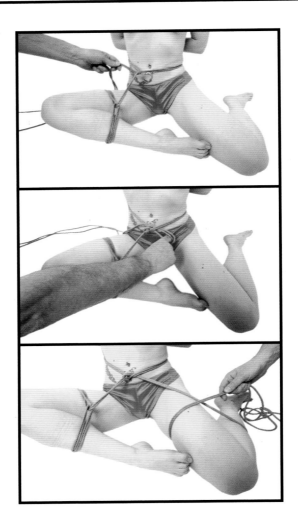

After you've wrapped the rope around the waist once, create a "tension loop" following the method detailed in chapter 3. Bring the rope to the other leg and wrap it once as you create a new tension point between the thigh and the ankle.

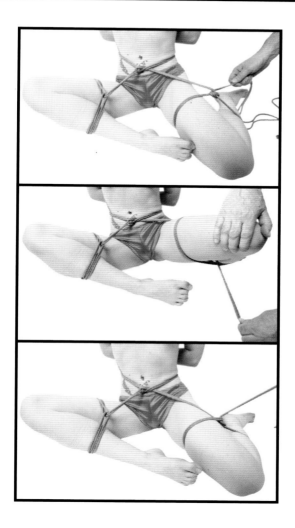

Secure the rope underneath, then bring the rope back to the tension point. In this version, I chose to wrap the rope twice around the first leg without securing it underneath. Next, I decided to wrap it once around the second leg while securing it this time. This is why it's always a good idea to leave room for improvisation. You'll always have to make decisions as you go along that are determined by the whole of your work, as well as from a practical point of view, depending on the remaining length of your rope. All of these factors combine to make your Shibari work unique.

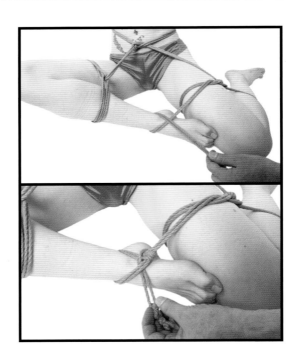

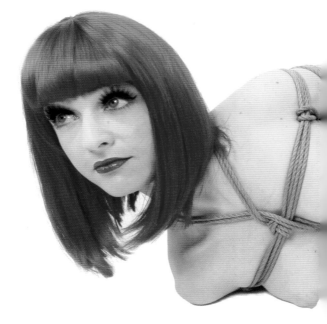

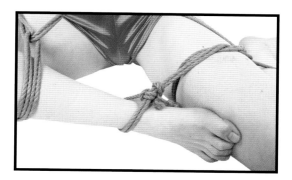

Finish the piece on the foot with a "tension loop" and an overhand knot.

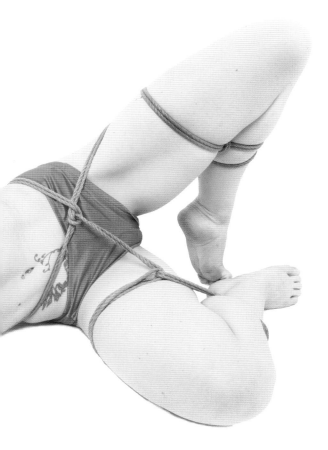

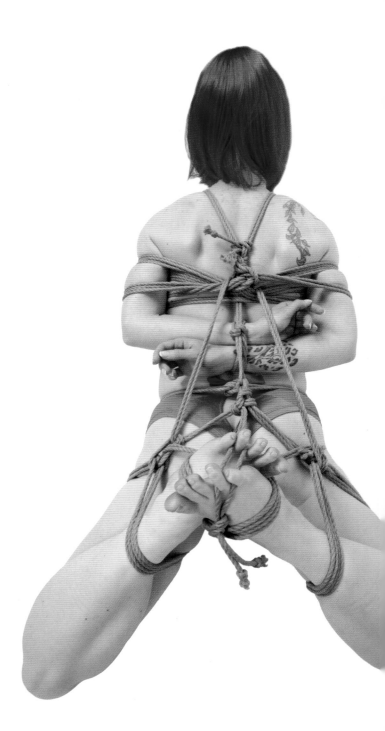

Hogtie

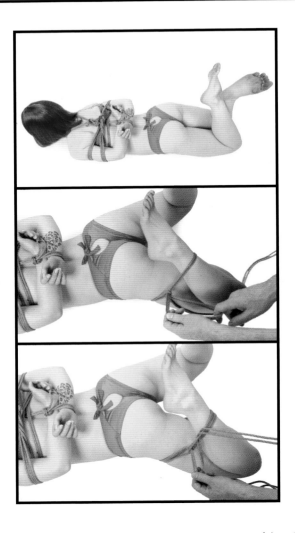

The hogtie is a classic in Shibari, and it's a strong, powerful method of restraint. To create a hogtie, we'll start the work at the chest with the arms put into bondage.

Have the model lie on her stomach.

Start with a lark's head on the folded leg.

Wrap the rope a second time after adjusting the counter-tension.

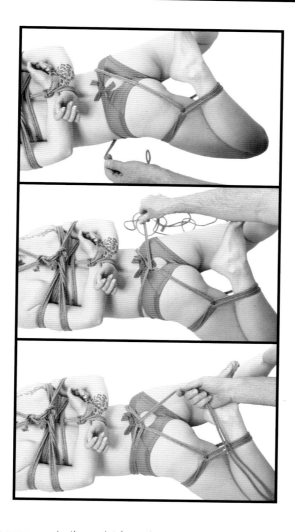

Bring the rope up to the waist from the opposite direction.
Adjust the counter-tension and wrap the rope a second time.
Then bring the rope down to the other leg.

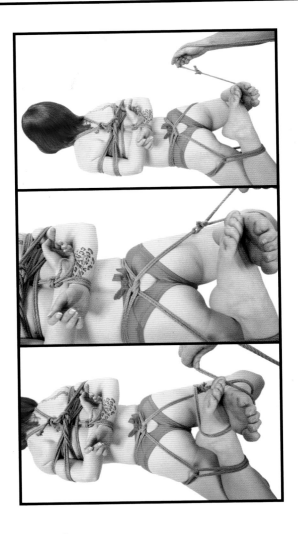

Extend your rope if necessary.

Wrap it twice as you did on the first leg, then bring the rope up to the feet.

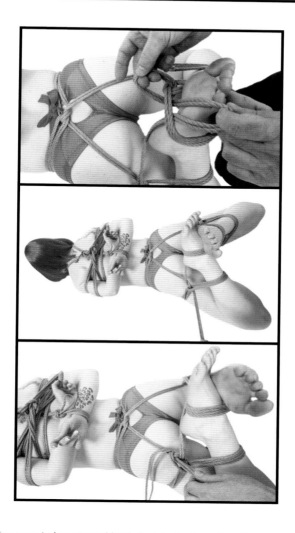

Wrap the rope twice around both feet to tie them together.
Tie an overhand knot, and then bring the rope back in tension to the binding point on the left leg in order to balance your work.
Tie another overhand knot here.

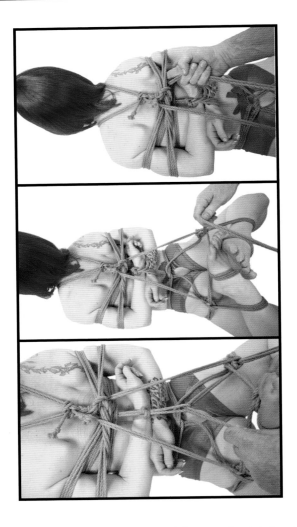

Adjust all the back wraps to get the model's upper body in tension with her legs.

Adjust on the right leg at the tension point, then apply an equal tension to the other leg.

Adjust the bight on the wrists.

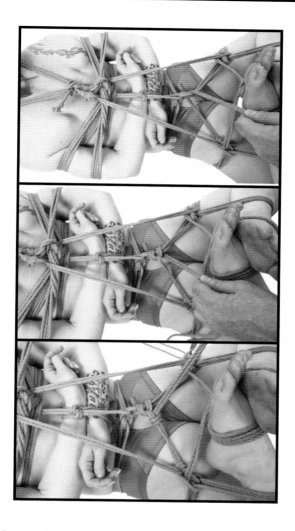

Now adjust on the left leg.

The tension you just added will have caused the ropes running between her waist and legs to become loose. So now you'll need to reduce slack by adjusting tension with the other ropes.

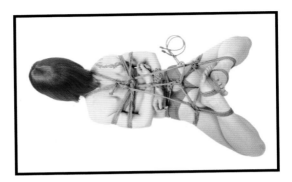

Finish the piece with an overhand knot.

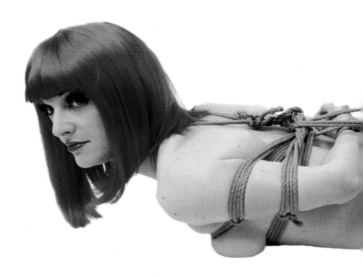

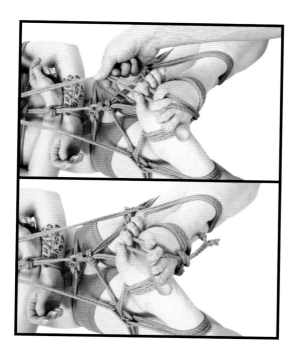

To use the excess rope, choose a part body part according to the remaining length. As shown here, the rope runs between the toes and is completed with a final knot.

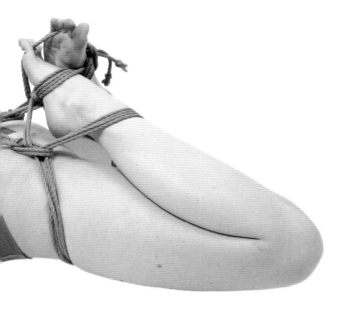

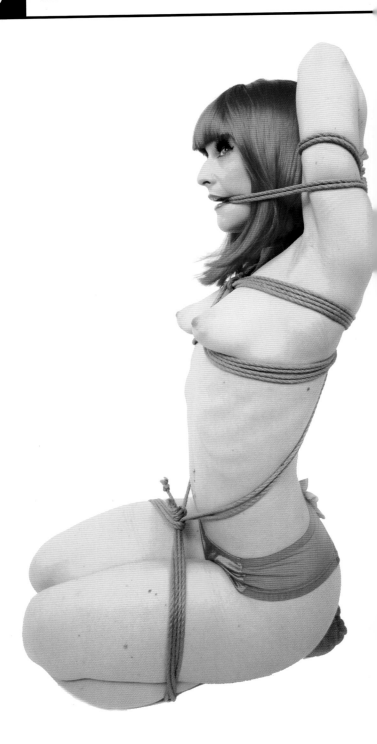

Arms behind head

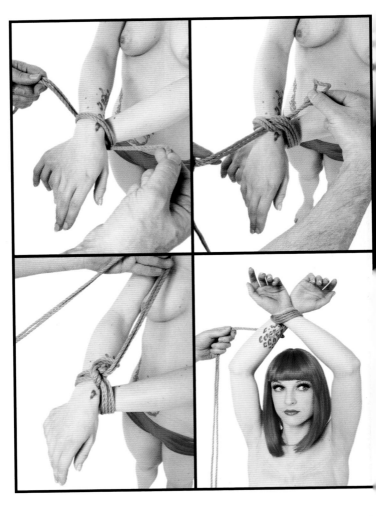

Start with the model's hands in front and wrap the rope twice around her wrists.

Tie a square knot while making sure there's a two-finger space left.

Now have your model raise her arms and cross her wrists behind her head.

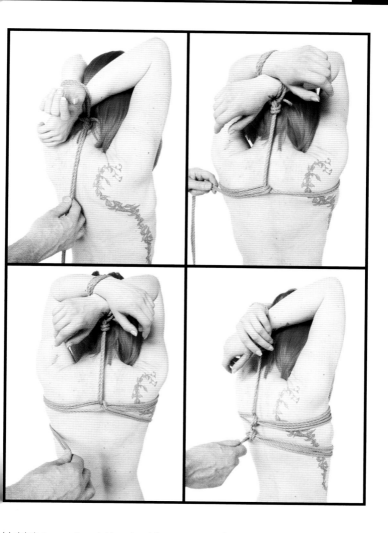

Hold the rope in mid-back while you wrap the rope around once above the breasts, then adjust the counter-tension.

Wrap the rope a second time, and again the same way under the breasts.

Wrap the rope twice, and cinch it with an overhand knot.

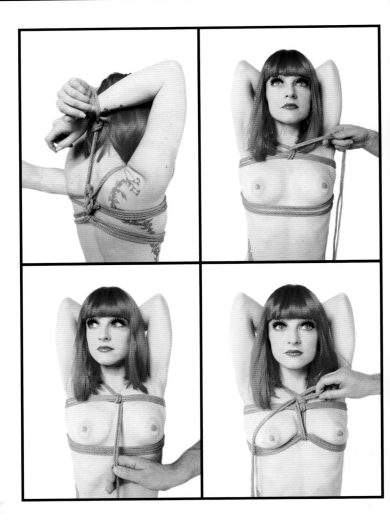

Create the first shoulder strap and create a coil of rope (the "tension loop") in front.

Choose the lower wrap; tuck the rope under the first shoulder strap and give it tension.

Return to the back as you create the second shoulder strap.

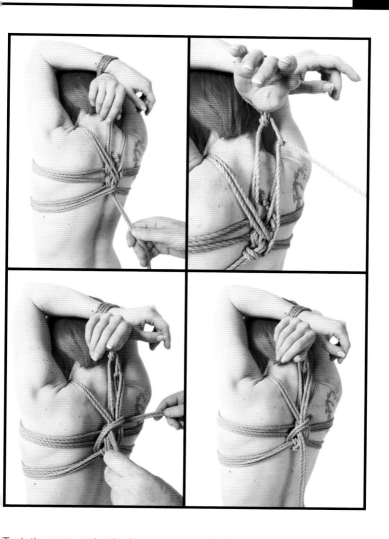

Tuck the rope under the lower wrap behind the back.
Use the bight on the wrists and give it tension.
Finish this section with an overhand knot.

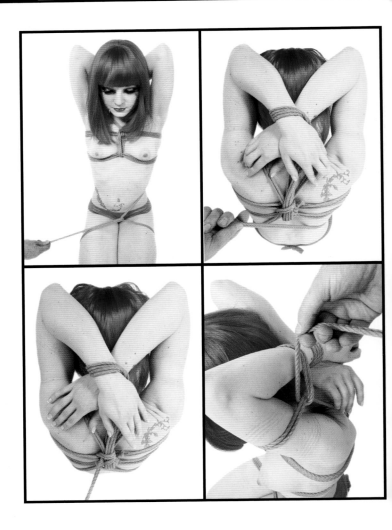

Move on to the next rope if necessary.

With the model in a kneeling position, bring the rope to her waist and wrap it around the legs a first time while positioning the counter-tension point in the middle.

Wrap the rope a second time.

Bring the rope up the other side and tie an overhand knot behind the back.

For the forearms, wrap the rope once here, and always select a tension point between the two parts of the arm.

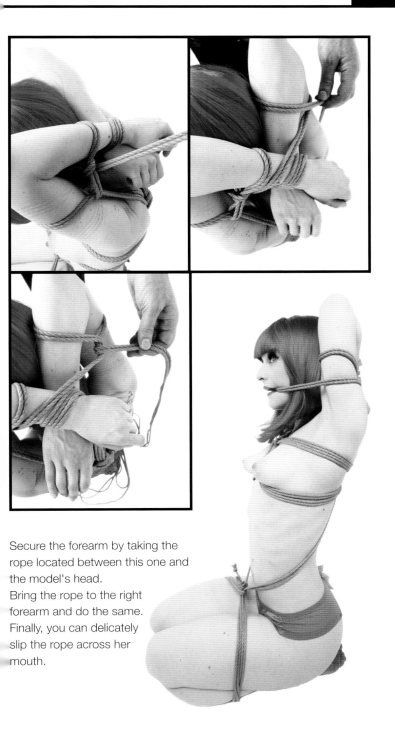

Secure the forearm by taking the
rope located between this one and
the model's head.
Bring the rope to the right
forearm and do the same.
Finally, you can delicately
slip the rope across her
mouth.

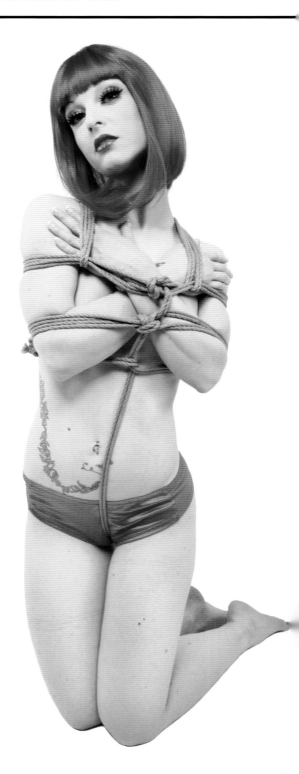

Hands crossed on chest

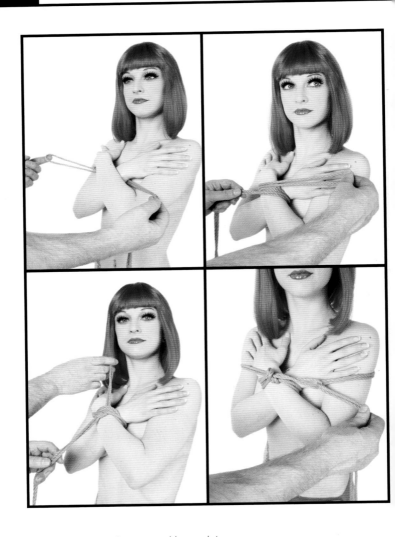

Wrap the rope twice around her wrists.
Use the whole wrap to tie a square knot.
Wrap the rope around the body and the wrists, then adjust the counter-tension through the bight on the wrists.

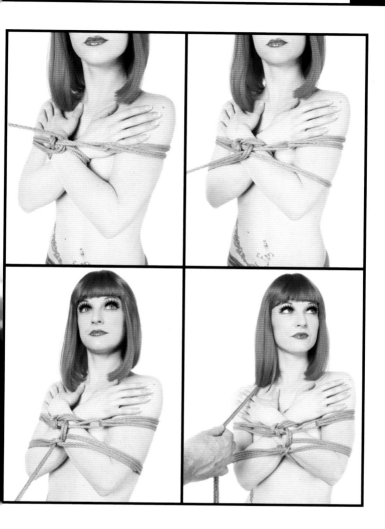

Wrap the rope a second time. Adjust the tension, this time on the wrists. Bring the rope around her body a little lower in the opposite direction, wrapped twice, closer to the elbows. Finish this part with an overhand knot. Bring the rope behind her back by passing it under the elbow and create the first shoulder strap as you return to the front.

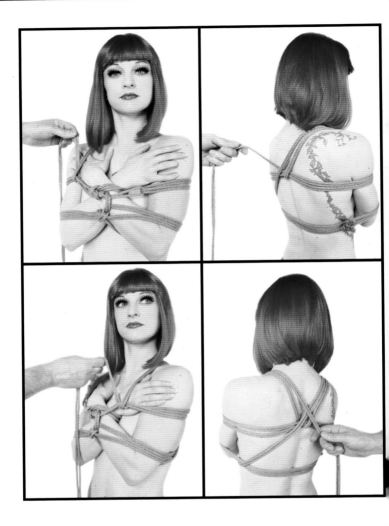

Take the wraps around the body and apply tension upward as you return to her back.

Tuck the rope through the back wraps once more, and return to the front to take the other side.

Then return to the back.

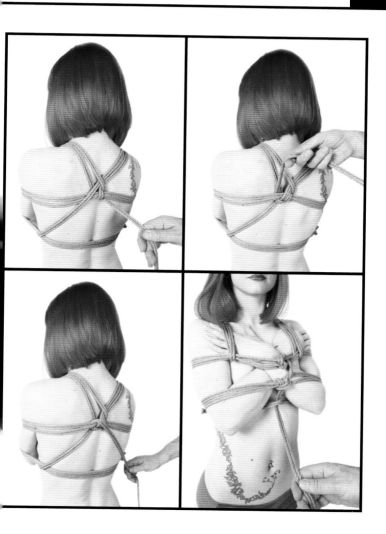

Applying tension behind the back, bring the rope back around to the front by passing it under the elbow and adjust the tension on the other rope on the opposite side.

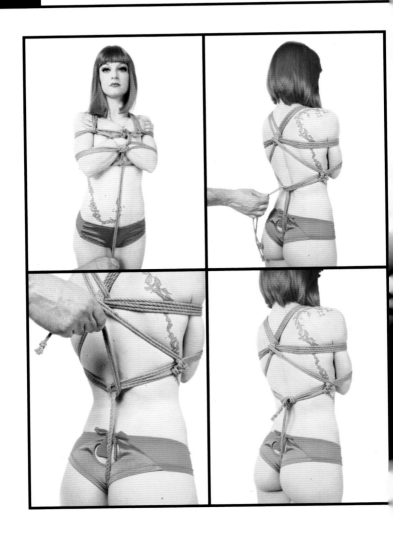

Bring the rope down between her legs.
Adjust the tension on the lower wrap in mid-back a last time.
Finish the piece with an overhand knot.

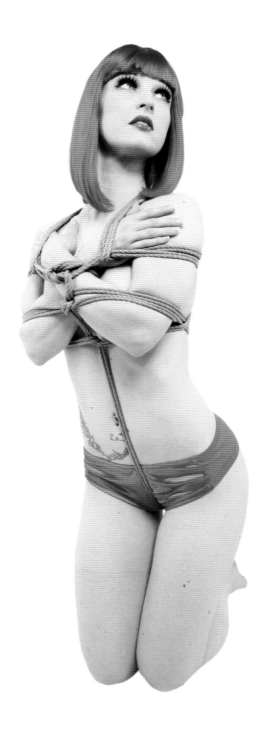

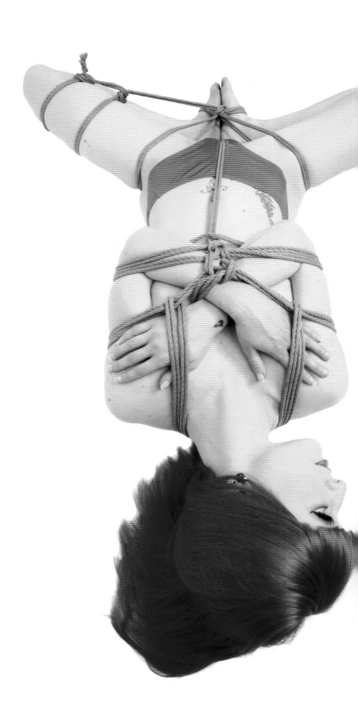

Finishing work on the legs

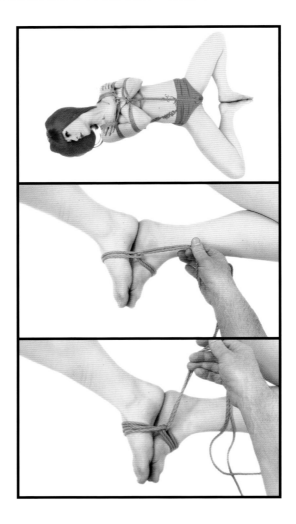

Position your model with her legs folded open, with the soles of her feet facing together.

Start with a lark's head.

Wrap the rope a second time in counter-tension.

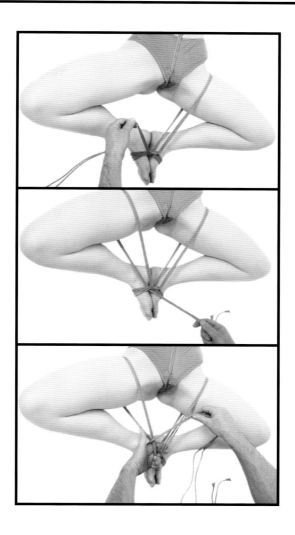

ake Wrap the leg at the upper thigh to maintain the restraint position.
3ring the rope back through the middle point on the feet, then do the
ame on the other leg. Cinch it with an overhand knot while you take all
ne ropes using your left hand.

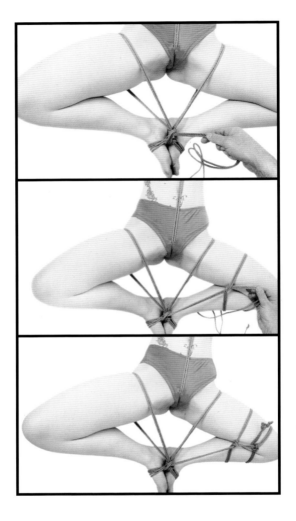

Bring the rest of the rope to one thigh. Wrap it once and bring it to the knee by using the "tension loop". Wrap the rope once more here in order to finish it, and cinch.

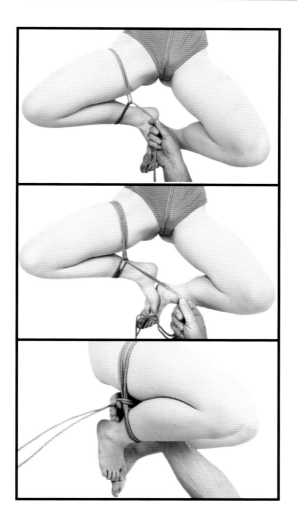

For the variant, start with a lark's head on the folded leg.
Wrap the rope a second time as you adjust its tension in the middle.
Secure it by passing the rope between the two parts of the leg.

The aim is to cinch the leg apart from the rest of your piece, so you must use the whole length in one go, doing so as aesthetically as possible.

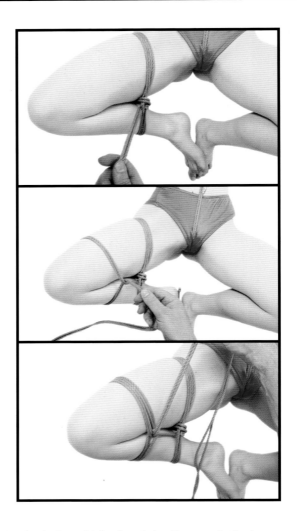

Adjust tension in the middle, then bring the rope to the knee.
Wrap the rope a first time, adjust in counter-tension, then wrap the rope
a second time.

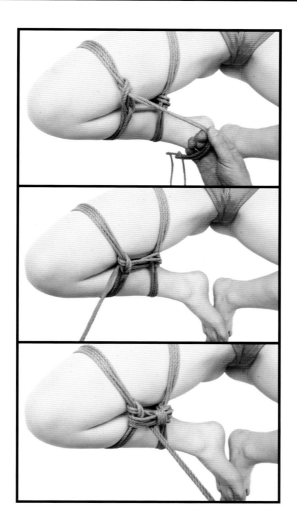

Tie an overhand knot, then wrap the rope between the two parts that fit the leg tightly two or three times, depending on the length you have. Finish this part by wrapping the rope around the whole tie you just made. Tie a last overhand knot.

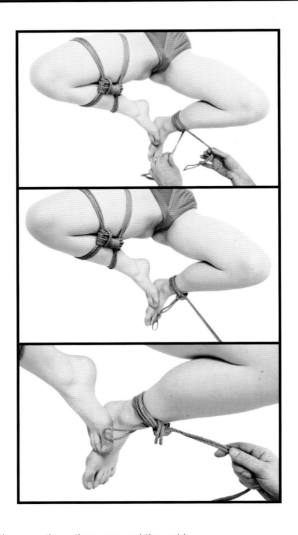

Wrap the rope three times around the ankle.

Tie a square knot with the entire wrap.

Using the whole wrap a second time, tie another knot.

Taking it a second time allows you to restrict the ropes from sliding, and to avoid cutting off the blood circulation.

This is particularly important for suspensions.

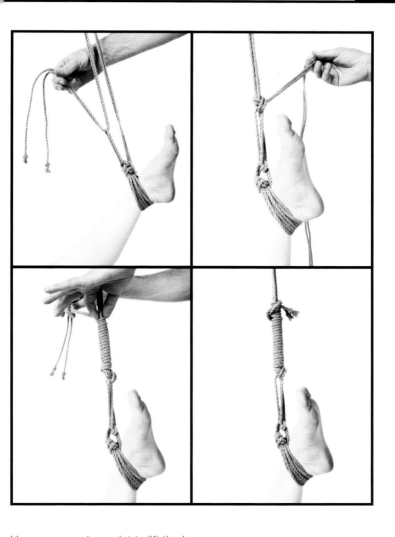

Use a suspension point to lift the leg.

Use the bight on the ankle; cinch it with an overhand knot.

Finish the rest of the rope by winding it up, and a final overhand knot.

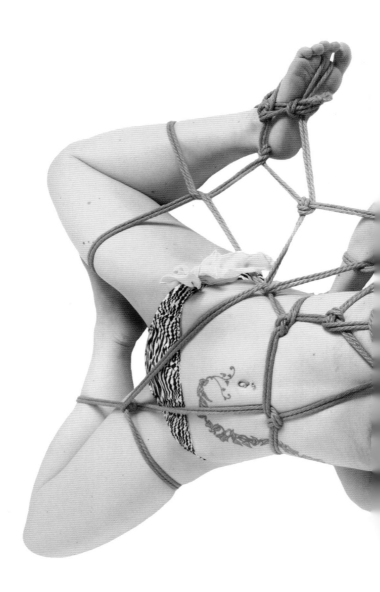

Floor improvisation

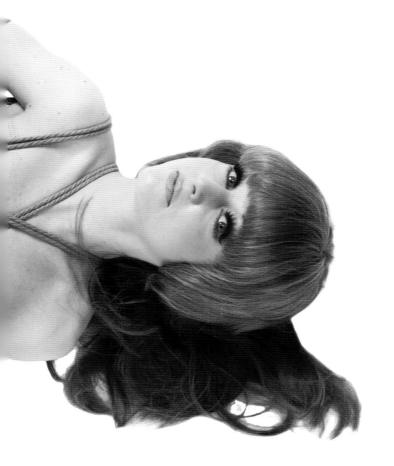

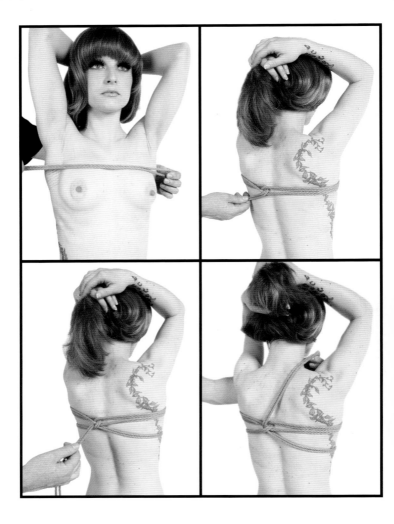

Place the rope above the breasts and create a lark's head behind the back.

Wrap the rope again above, then once below, always using the tension and counter-tension method.

Bring the rope up to her neck to create the first shoulder strap.

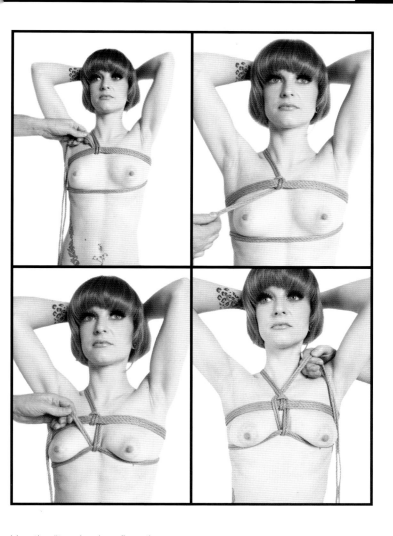

Use the "tension loop" on the upper wrap.
Run it under the lower wrap to give it tension.
Then tuck the rope under the first shoulder strap and create a second
one to balance the middle tension.

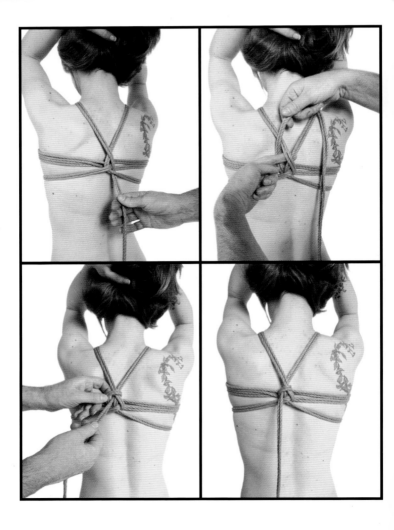

Bring the rope back to the starting point in mid-back as you pass under the ropes.

Finish this section with an overhand knot on the shoulder straps.

Drop the excess rope for the moment; you will use it afterwards.

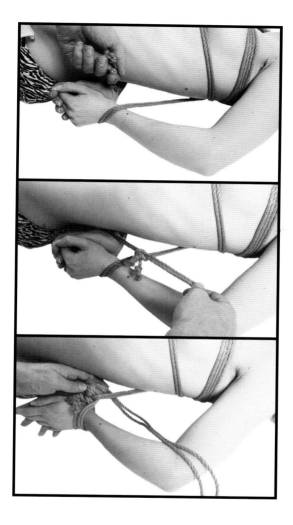

Position your model on the floor, lying on her back, with her hands slightly aside.

Wrap the rope around the hands twice, while extending your rope if necessary.

Using the whole wrap on the wrist, tie an overhand knot.

Use the technique from chapter 2 to avoid cutting off her circulation.

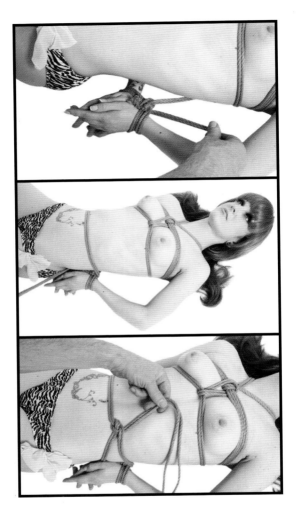

Apply tension upward, then wrap the rope around her waist.
Bring this wind around the waist with its "tension loop" up to the chest

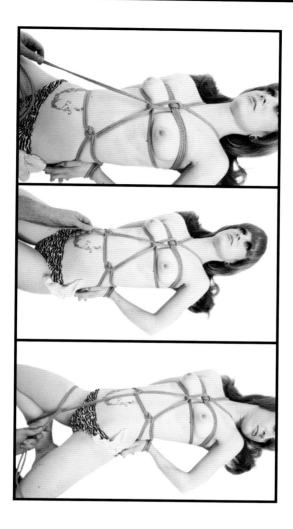

Tuck the rope through the loop on the chest.
Apply tension by taking the wind around the waist on the other side, always using the "tension loop".
Bring the rope down to her thigh and wrap it around once. Bring the rope up to the wind located between the wrists and the waist.

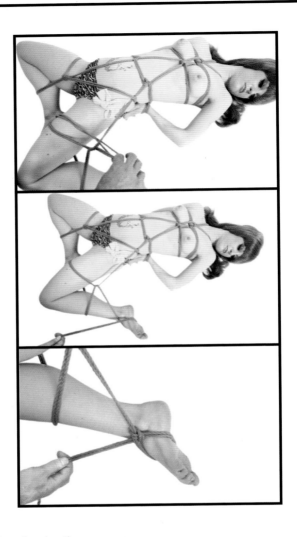

Bind the other leg the same way.

Finish this part by wrapping the rope once around the foot using the "tension loop".

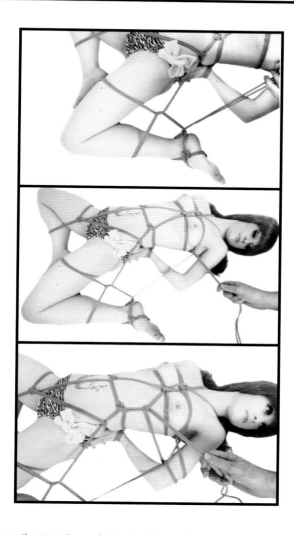

Create another tension point behind the ankle.

Bring the rope up to the upper wrap on the chest.

Wrap the rope once around the arm, then again a little lower, while utilizing the rope that went up the chest.

Apply tension on the rope between her waist and breasts.

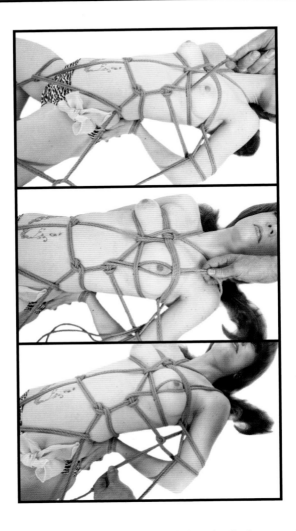

Bring the rope over her breast as you tuck it under the lower and upper wraps on the chest.

Bring the rope over the shoulder.

Take the rope between the elbow and the body with a "tension loop".

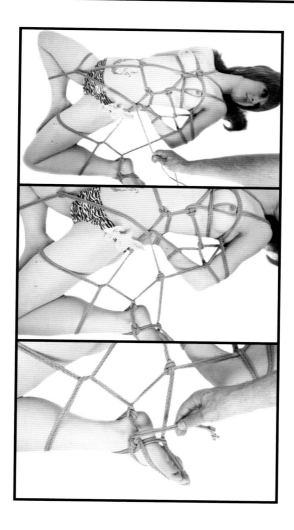

Wrap the rope once around the wrist and bring the rope back in tension using the rope running along the hip. Create a new "tension loop" on the rope between the elbow and the foot. Tuck this rope under the one located at the arch of the foot, then run it between the toes. Adjust the tension on the ankle then finish the piece with an overhand knot.

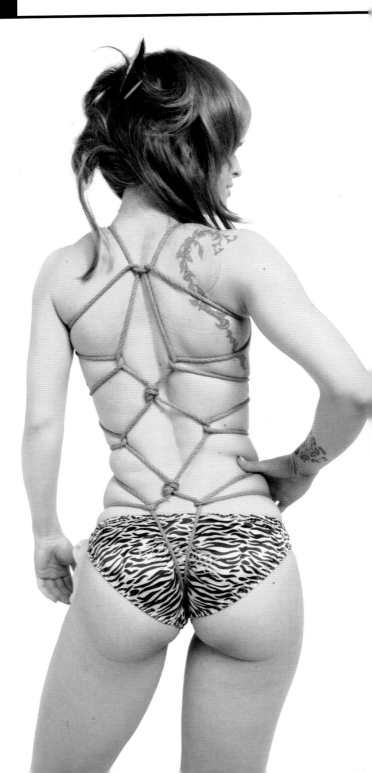

Karada

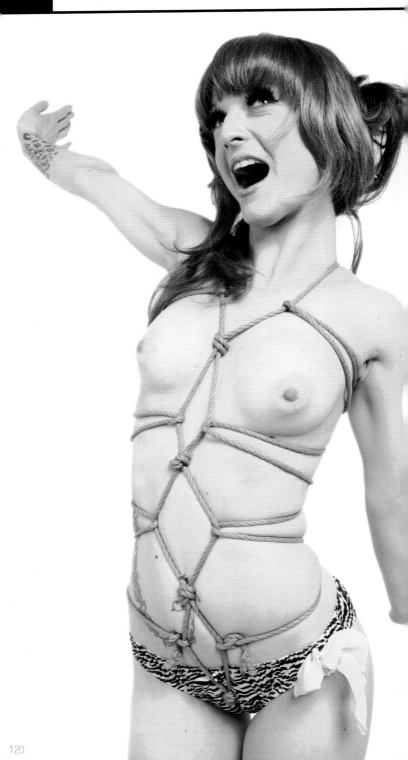

Karada
for a base

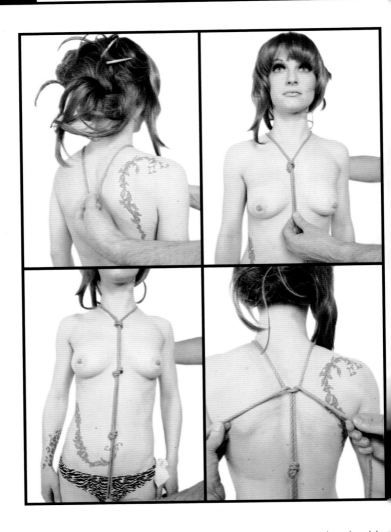

Start at the rope's center point while holding it between the shoulder blades, level with the armpits. Tie an overhand knot below the neck, a second one below the bust, then a third one midway between the crotch and bust. Run the rope down between her legs and bring it up along the back. Tie another knot at waist level, then a final one between the waist and starting point. Get the rope in tension by splitting its ends apart.

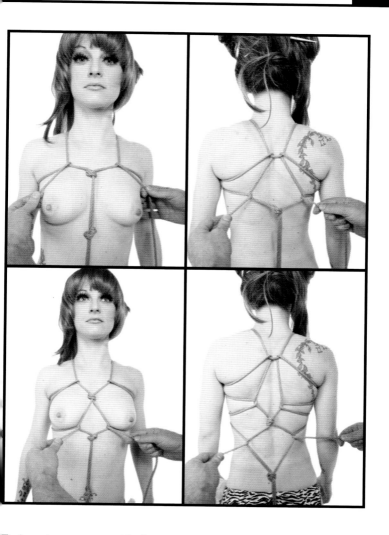

Tuck each rope symmetrically under the "necklace". Apply tension, then return to the back to split the rope's ends apart. Do the same on the front, and repeat. Finish each rope separately with an overhand knot.

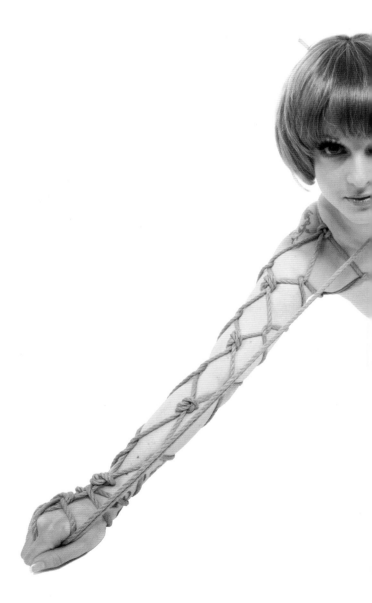

Karada
on the arm

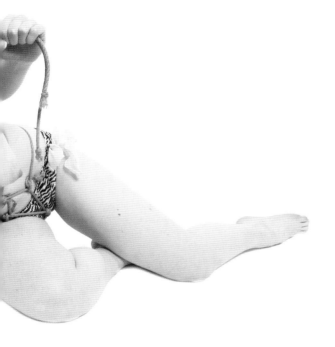

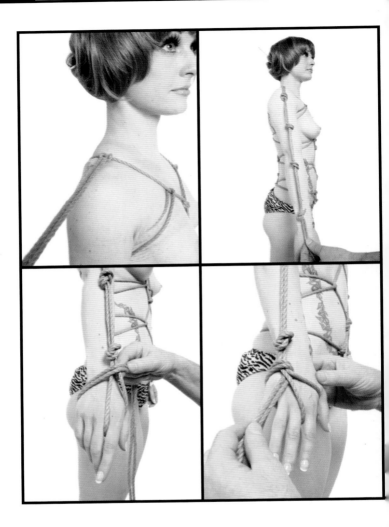

Begin with a lark's head using the previous Karada on the shoulder.
Tie a series of four regularly-spaced knots.
Split the rope ends around her index finger, wrap the rope around the
wrist, and adjust its tension.

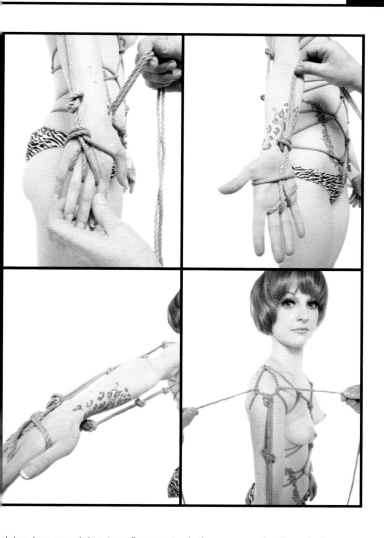

Using her remaining two fingers, tuck the rope under the wind across the palm of her hand, and then continue the series of knots.
Use the ropes of the previous Karada below the armpit.
Split the ends apart and apply tension as you start on the shoulder.

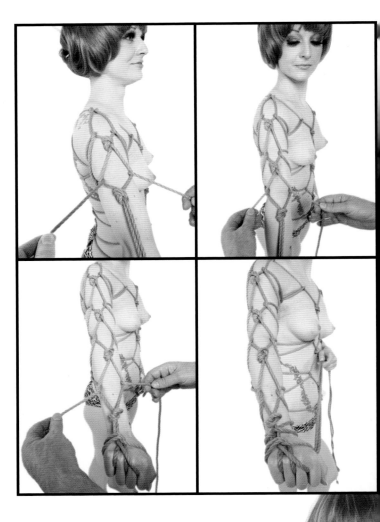

Continue this technique all the way to the wrist.

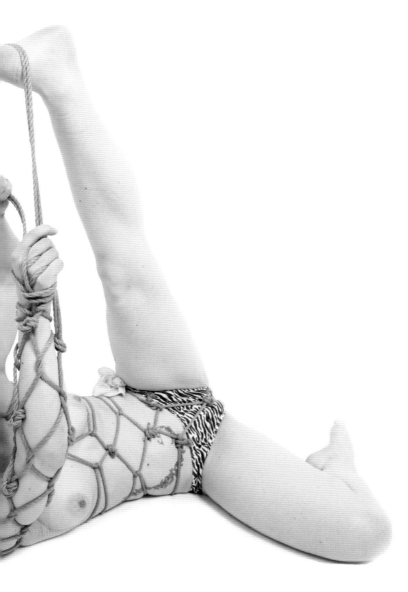

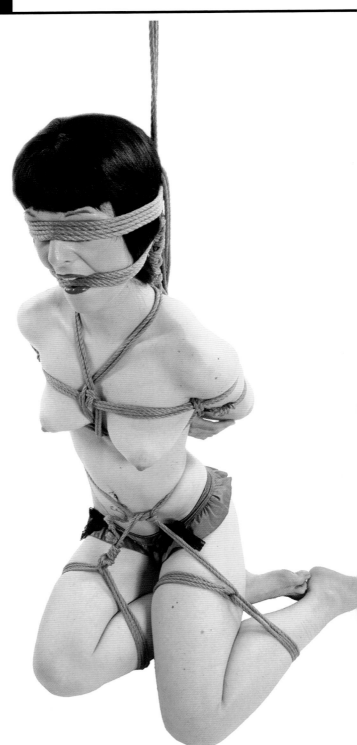

Sitting with eyes and mouth bound

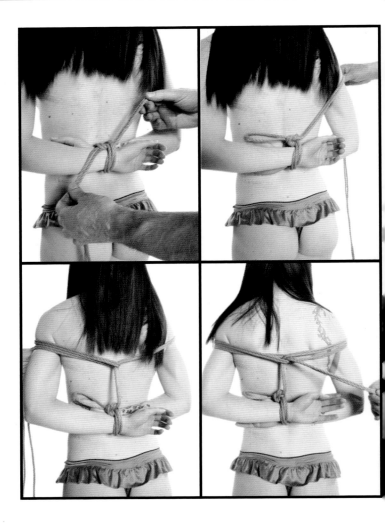

Commencer par deux tours sur les poignets, sans bloquer la circulation.
Remonter au milieu du dos, puis faire deux tours en dessus de poitrine en reprenant les tensions.

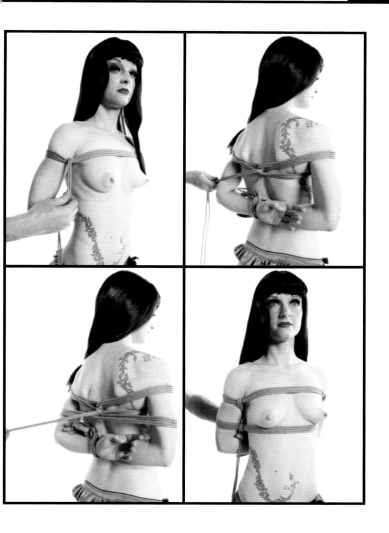

Secure the rope by tucking it from top to bottom on both sides.
Wrap the rope twice below the breasts, securing it again.

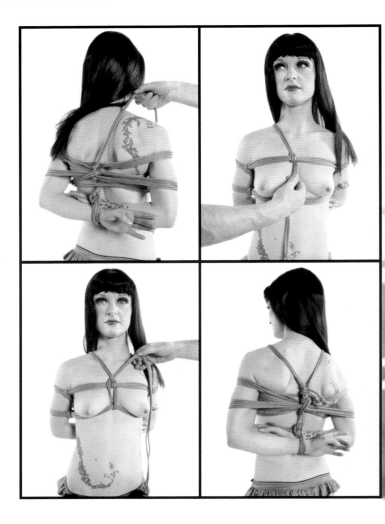

Adjust the counter-tension in mid-back and bring the rope over her shoulder create the first strap.

Create a "tension loop" on the upper wrap. Tuck the rope under the lower wrap and create the second shoulder strap. Be sure to pass it under the first one, against the tension point.

Cinch the end of the rope behind her back.

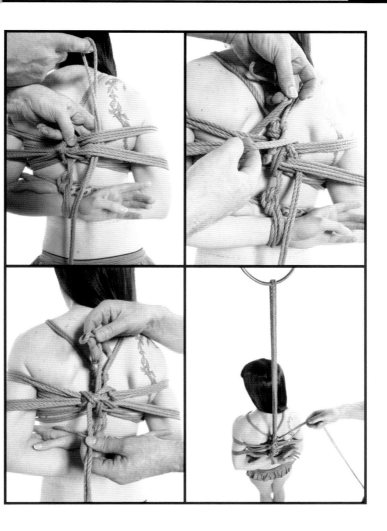

Using a new rope, create a figure eight that begins under the right-side ropes, working from bottom to top. Then once again from bottom to top over the left ropes.

Take all the ropes forming the figure eight and tie a square knot while leaving a long bight.

Bring the rope up to the suspension point then bring it back down and take the bight.

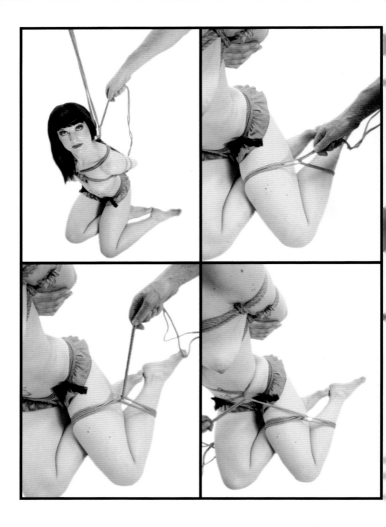

Have your model sit down so you can cinch the retaining rope toward the suspension point.

Create a lark's head on the folded leg and wrap the rope twice.

Bring the rope around her waist, then down around the other leg.

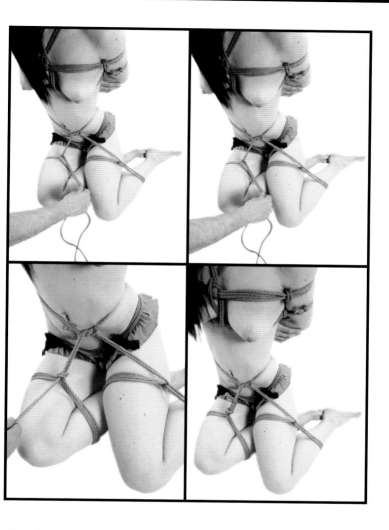

Wrap the rope around the other leg twice, applying counter-tension at each wind.
Tie an overhand knot, then finish your rope by winding it up.

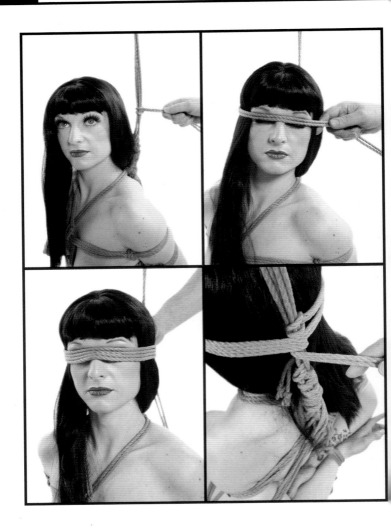

On the rope that goes to the suspension point, use a new piece of rope and create a lark's head at the model's eye-level.
Wrap the rope very gently over her eyes twice, adjusting the tension between the two.

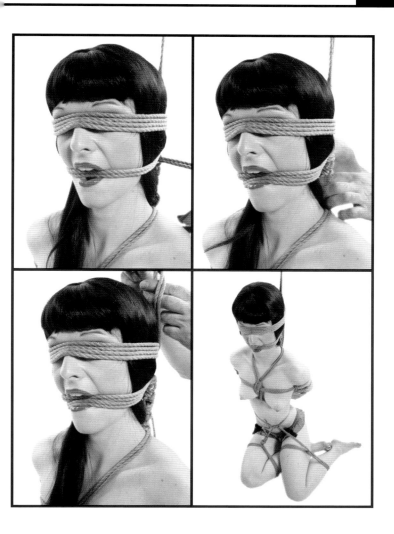

Wrap the rope around her head and carefully between her lips (to open her mouth) twice. You'll finish by cinching the rest of the rope.

It's extremely important that all the work on and around her head, face and neck must be done gently and with great care.

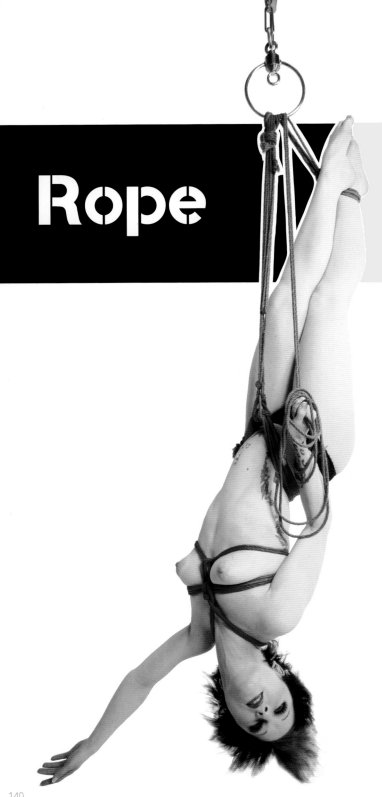

Rope

suspensions

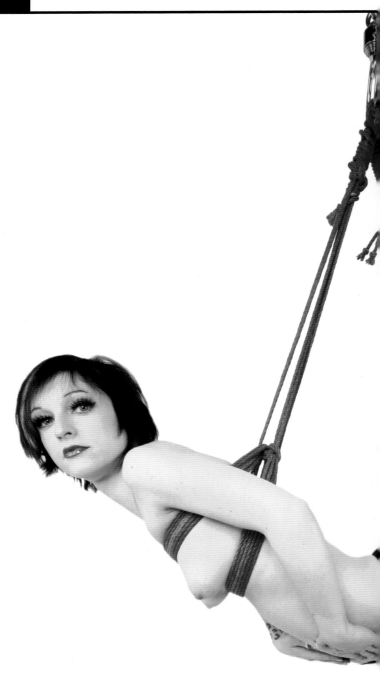

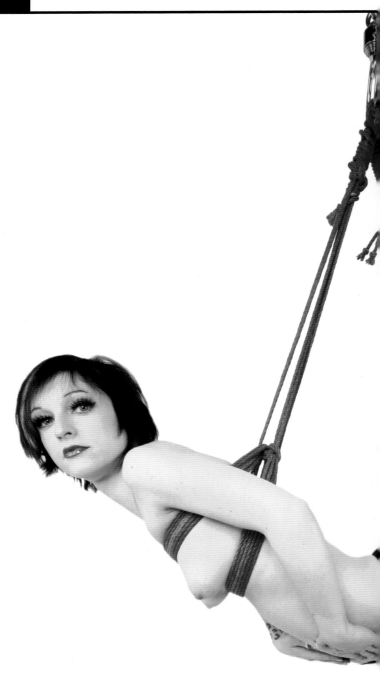

Back suspension

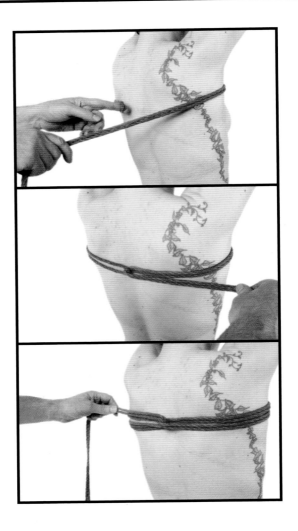

**Before you attempt any suspension Shibari,
re-read the "Safety and advice" section on page 17.**

Start above the breasts, and create a lark's head behind her back.
Adjust the tension and wrap the rope a second time.

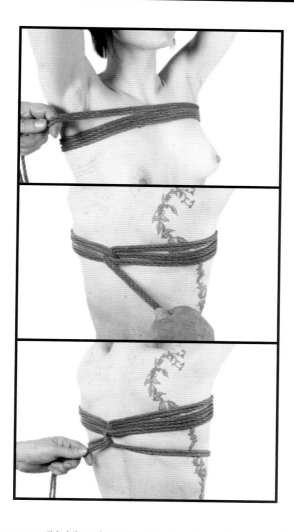

Wrap the rope a third time then adjust the tension and wrap again, below
the breasts.
Wrap the rope again and adjust the tension.

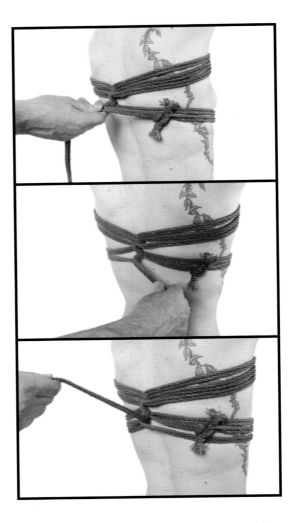

Wrap the rope under her breasts two more times (three total), repeating the technique.

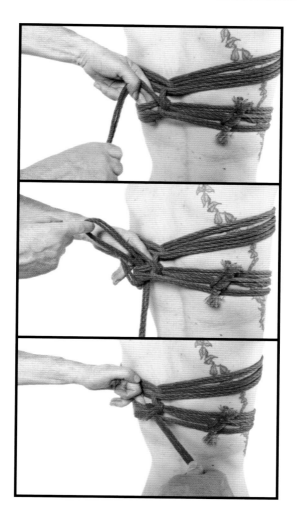

Finish this section with an overhand knot on the last three ropes of the lower wrap

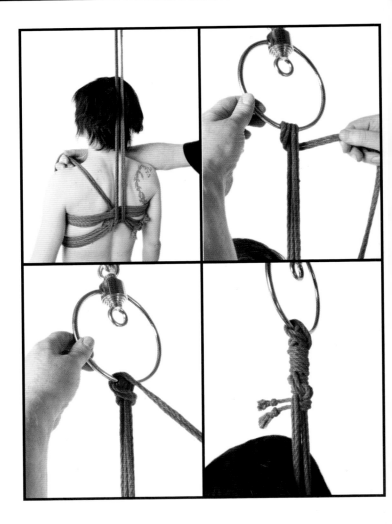

Run the rope through the suspension ring, then take all the back wraps and run the rope through the ring again.
Form a coil by going behind the ropes then up onto the ring.
Finish the rope by winding the remaining length all the way down, and cinch with a series of overhand knots.

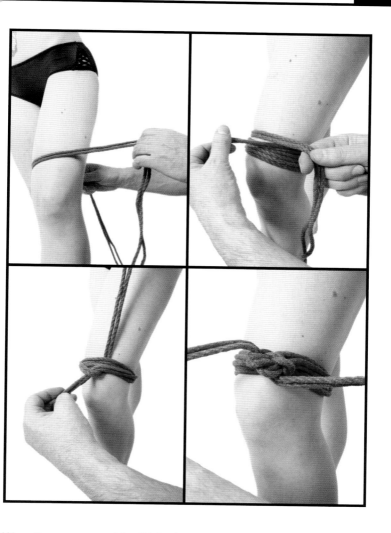

Wrap the rope around the thigh above the knee.
Wrap it three times as you adjust the length so there's a long bight left
and a two-finger space between the ropes and the leg.
Take the whole wrap and tie a square knot.

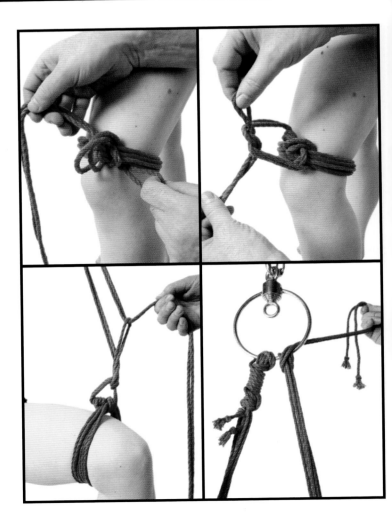

Using the whole wrap again, tie a second square knot.

Lift the leg up while running the rope through the suspension point and take the bight.

Bring the rope up onto the ring and form a coil as before.

Finish with an overhand knot after you've wound the rope down.

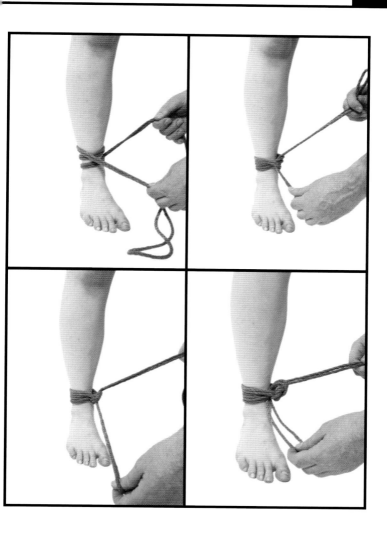

Wrap the rope three times around the ankle on the other leg.
Use the whole wrap to finish with a square knot while making sure you keep a long bight.

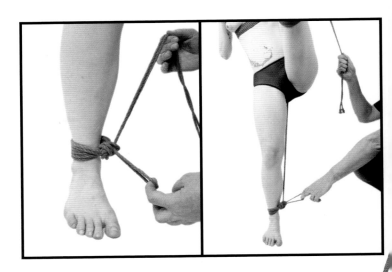

Get ready to lift the model up as you take the rope and the bight in your hands.
Run the rope through the ring and pull while lifting the leg up in order to take the bight.

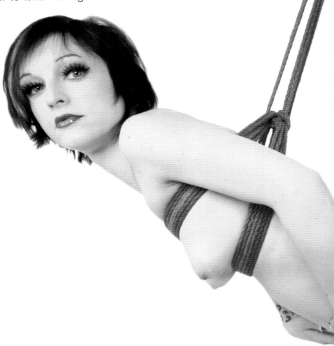

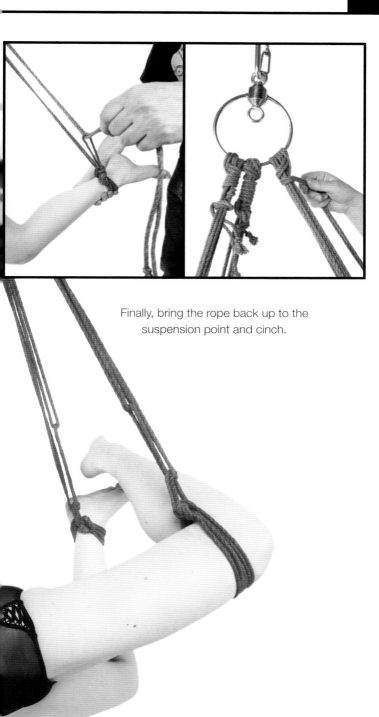

Finally, bring the rope back up to the suspension point and cinch.

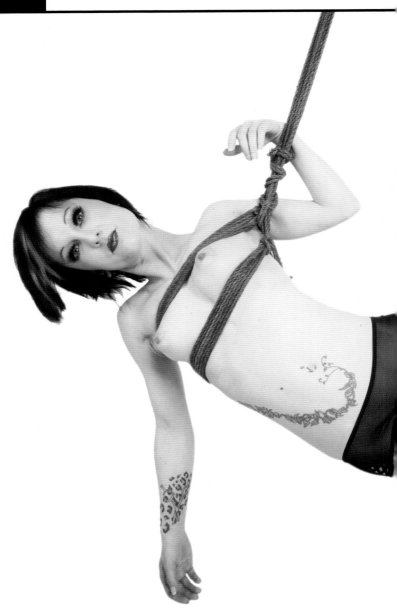

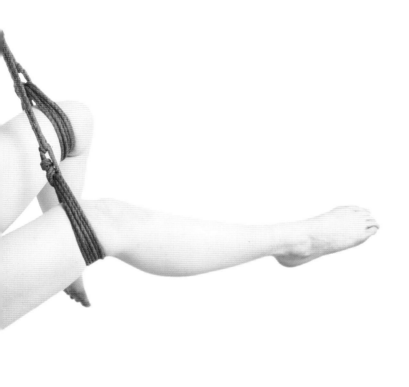

Side
suspension

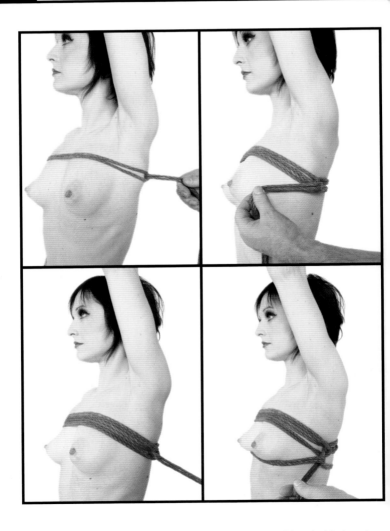

Wrap the rope once above the model's breasts with a lark's head on the side.
Wrap the rope two more times while adjusting the tension at every wind. Continue below the breasts.

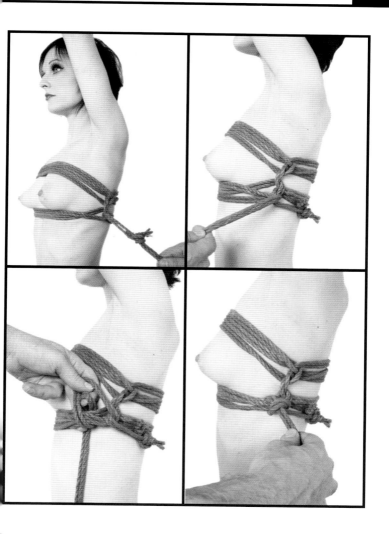

Wrap the rope three times, then take the whole lower wrap and cinch.

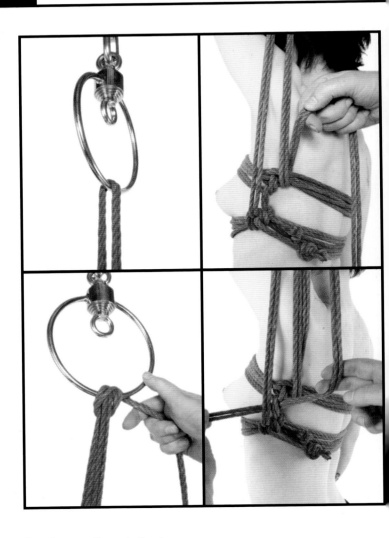

Run the rope through the ring.
Run it back under the whole upper wrap.
Bring the rope back up to the ring, then back down again and through
the ropes between the upper and lower wraps.

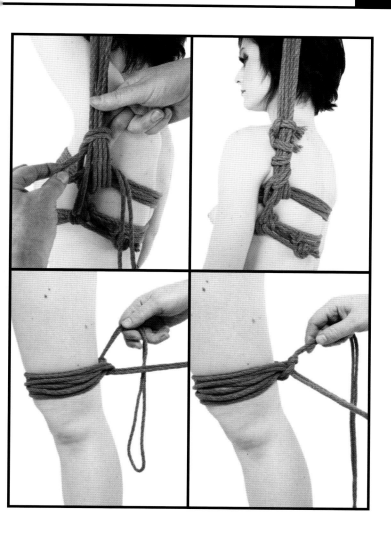

Finally, tie a series of overhand knots or wind the remaining length upward.

Wrap a new rope above the knee and proceed with the same technique as you did for the back suspension.

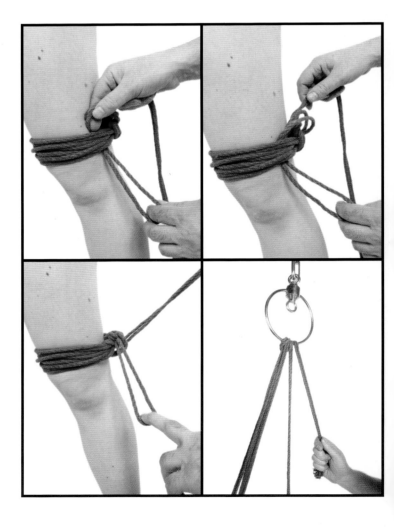

Double the knot.
Bring the rope up to the ring.

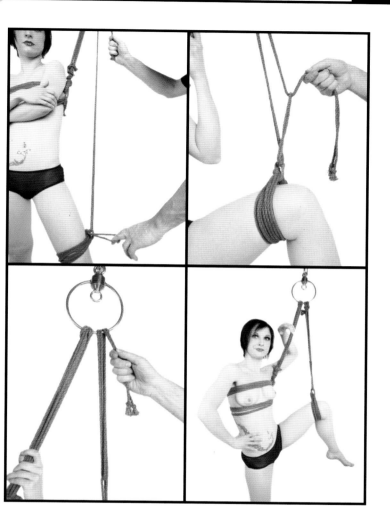

Lift the leg up and take the bight.
Bring the rope up to the ring and cinch.

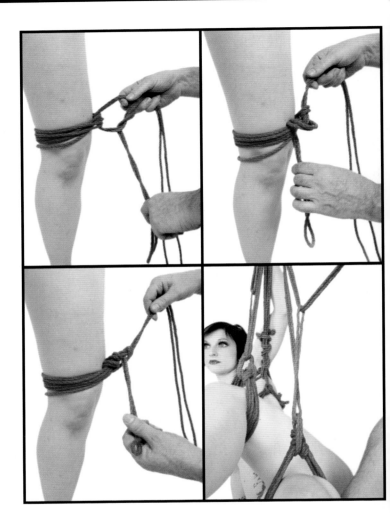

Wrap a new rope above the knee around the other leg, double the knot and lift the model up.

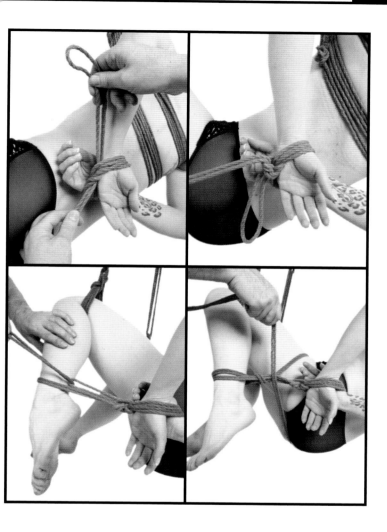

Next, you can bind her hands behind her back by wrapping the rope twice around her wrists and leaving a bight.

Wrap the rope once around the ankle. Take the bight then wrap the rope a second time around the ankle.

Finish the rope around the thigh then bring it up through the ring to cinch it.

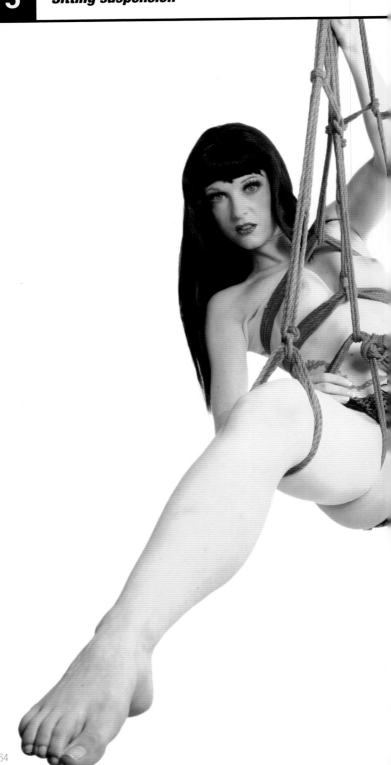

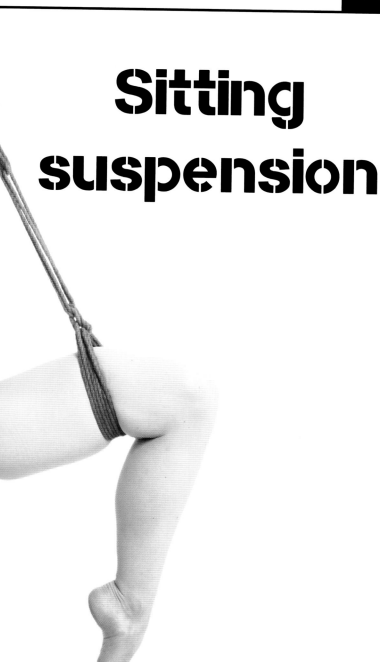

Sitting suspension

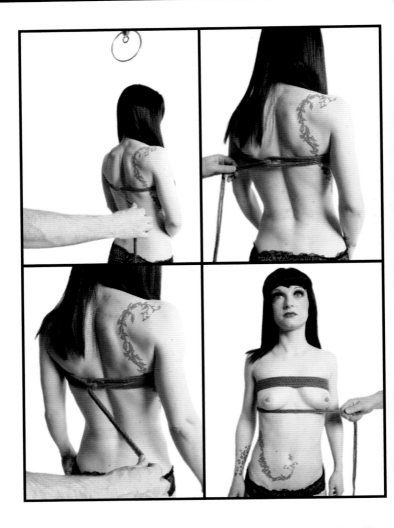

Start by running the rope above her breasts and make a lark's head behind her back.

Wrap the rope three times above her breasts and repeat three times below her breasts.

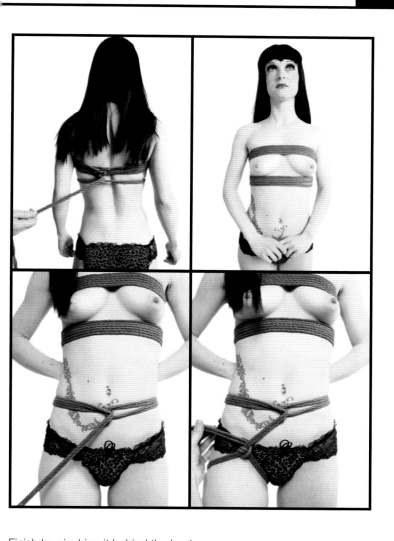

Finish by cinching it behind the back.

Wrap a new rope twice around her waist.

Bring that rope down to one thigh, wrap it once around and create a "tension loop".

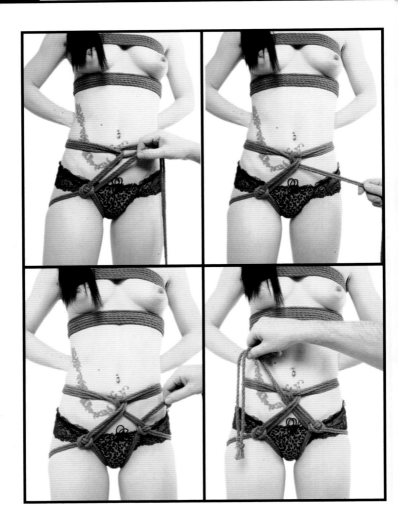

Bring the rope up to the middle point on her waist, and then back down to the other thigh, and repeat.

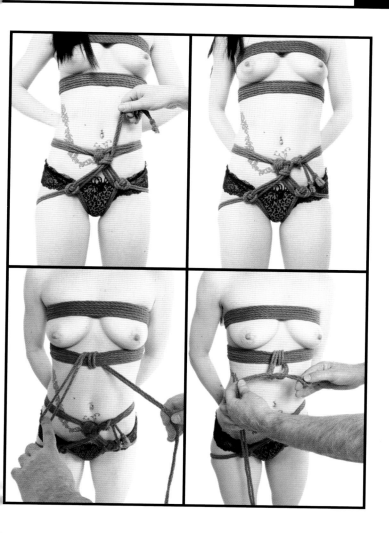

Tie an overhand knot at the middle point and get rid of the excess rope
by winding it up.

Coil a new rope twice over the lower wrap on the chest, then tie a square
knot while leaving a long bight.

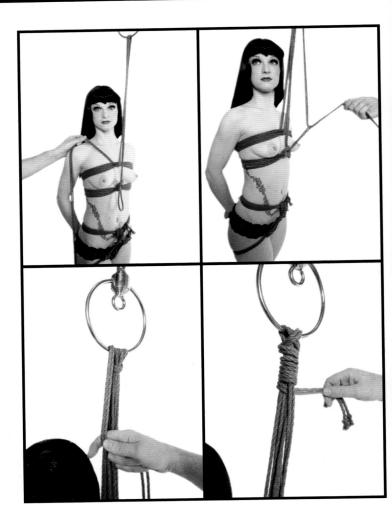

Bring the rope up to the ring then down through the upper wrap on the chest.

Bring the rope back up to the ring, then down again, and take the bight.

Bring the rope up to the ring a last time and finish.

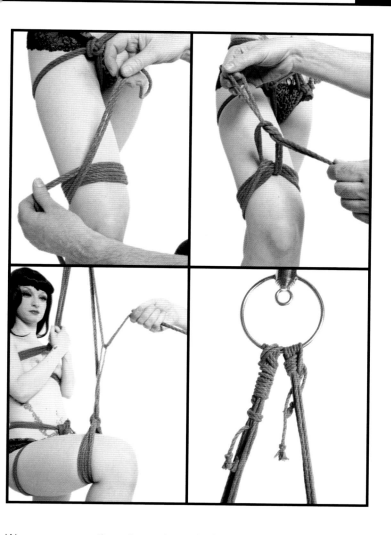

Wrap a new rope three times above the knee.
Tie a double knot, then lift the leg up and cinch the rope onto the ring.

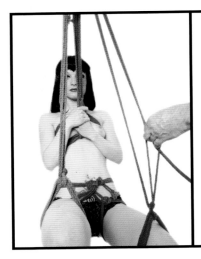 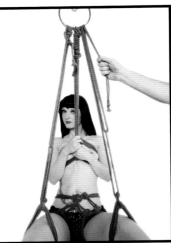

Do the same with the second leg.
With a new rope and a lark's head, take the
ropes on the waist and those going down the
thigh – do this on the side of the middle point.
Bring the rope up to the ring and back down
to anchor under the other side.
Return to the ring and cinch.

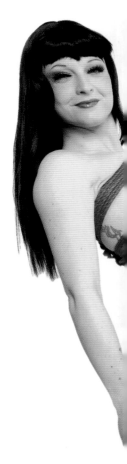

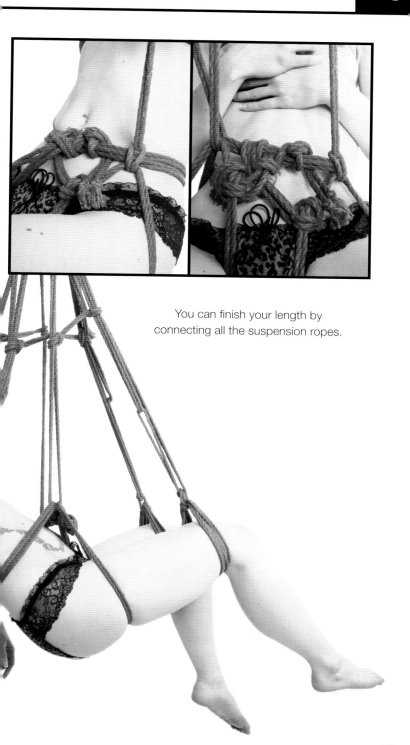

You can finish your length by connecting all the suspension ropes.

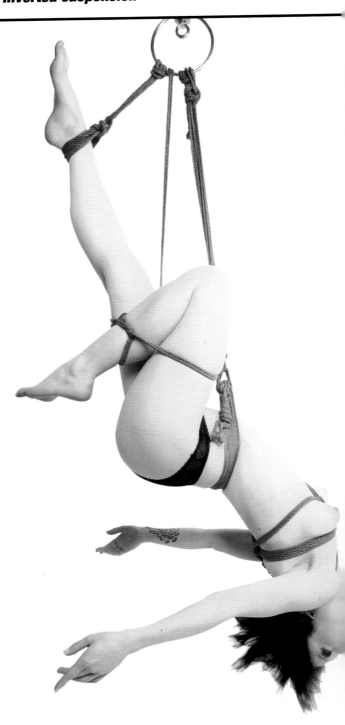

Inverted suspension

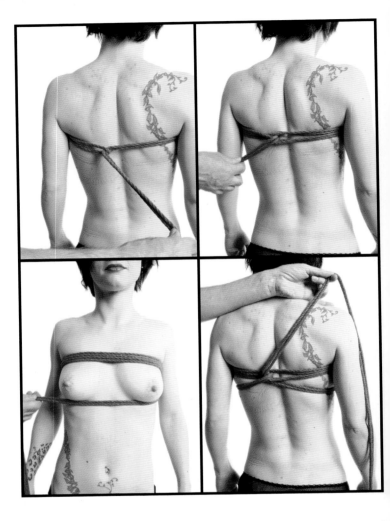

Start wrapping the rope once above the breasts and create a lark's head behind the back.

Wrap the rope twice above then once below the breasts.

Adjust the tension and create the first shoulder strap.

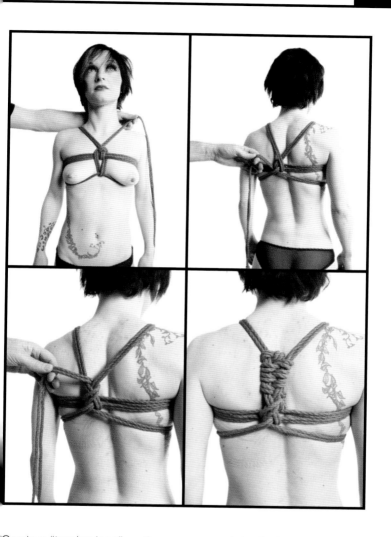

Create a "tension loop" on the upper wrap, take the lower wrap, then create the second shoulder strap after you've adjusted the opposite tension on the upper chest. Take the lower wrap behind the back and finish by winding the rope all the way up the shoulder straps, once underneath, once over.

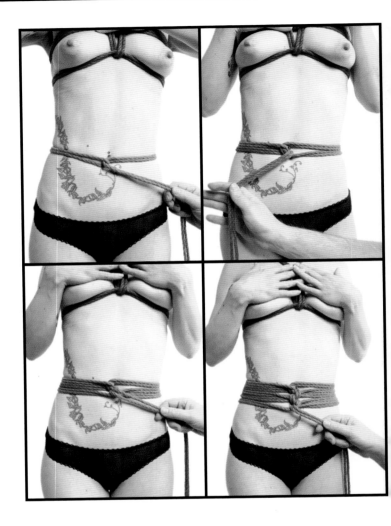

Start with a lark's head on the waist without tightening.
Wrap the rope all the way down while adjusting the tension at every coil
of the wind above.

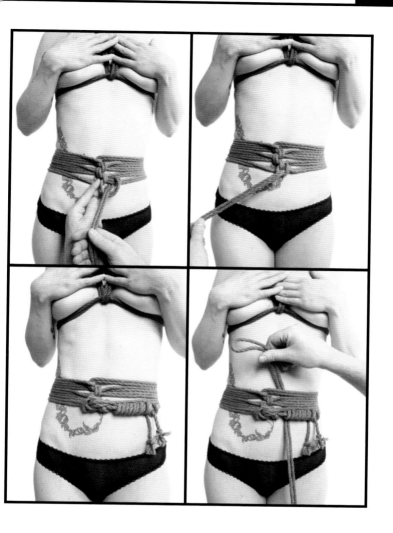

Finish with a double overhand knot and get rid of the excess rope by winding it up.

Tuck a new rope under the harness you just created.

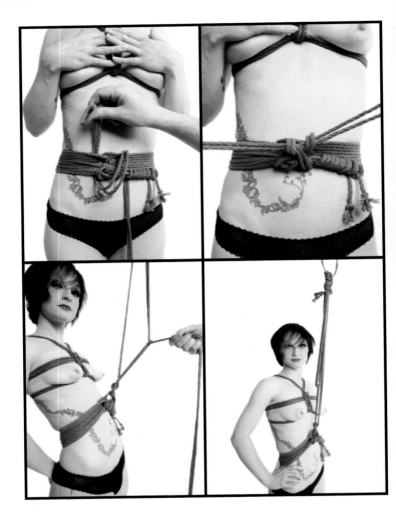

Tuck the rope under the harness a second time.
Take all the ropes that form the figure eight, tie a square knot and leave a bight.
Bring the rope up to the ring and cinch.

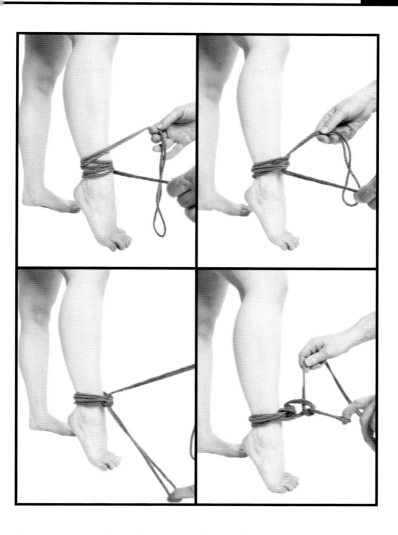

Wrap a new rope three times around one ankle.
Tie a square knot, then double it.

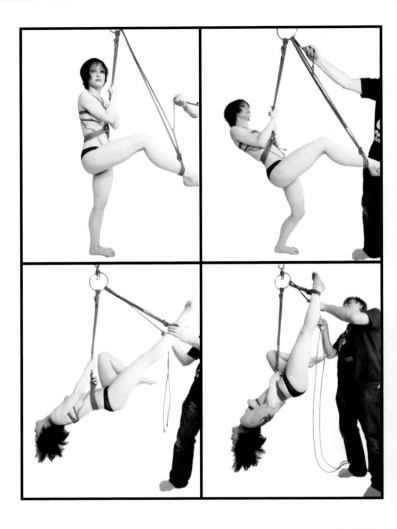

Bring the rope up to the ring then bring it back down and take the bight. Bring the rope back up to the ring and pull to topple the model over backwards, while she leans at the waist.

Coil the rope onto the ring to cinch it and bring the rope back down.

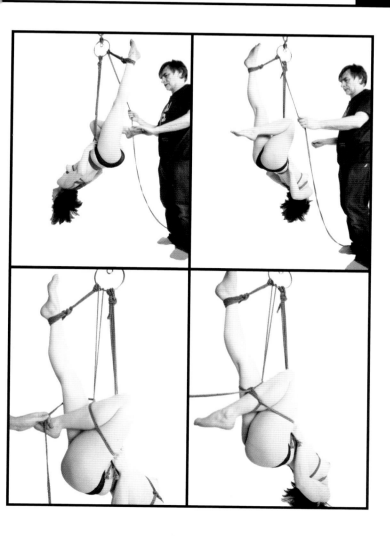

Wrap the rope once around the other leg, which must be folded, then wrap it once around the suspended leg; finish by adjusting the tension on the rope that runs around the folded leg.

Get rid of the remaining length by wrapping it once more around the suspended leg.

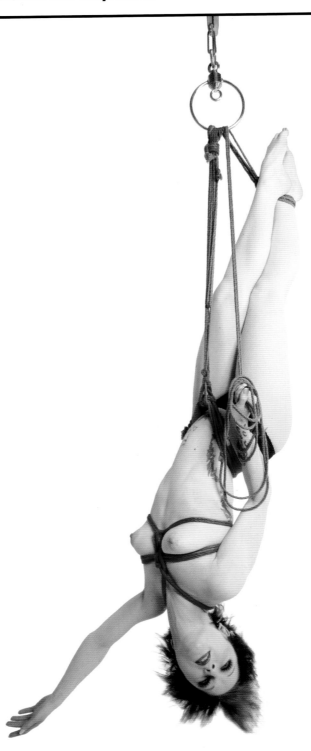

Inverted self-suspension

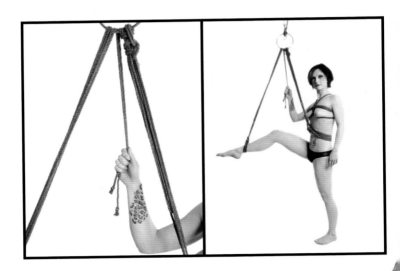

To perform a self-suspension, you only have to prepare the same base as in the previous chapter. The model will lift up her tied leg while giving an impetus to her body to topple over backwards.

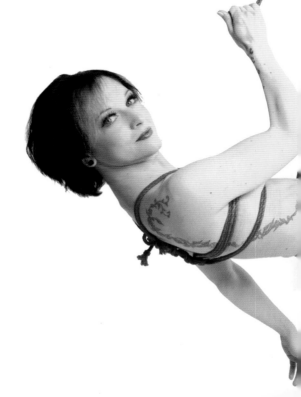

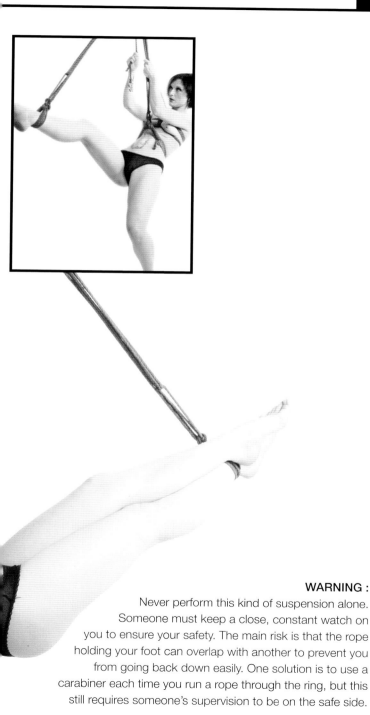

WARNING :
Never perform this kind of suspension alone.
Someone must keep a close, constant watch on
you to ensure your safety. The main risk is that the rope
holding your foot can overlap with another to prevent you
from going back down easily. One solution is to use a
carabiner each time you run a rope through the ring, but this
still requires someone's supervision to be on the safe side.

Bamboo cros suspension

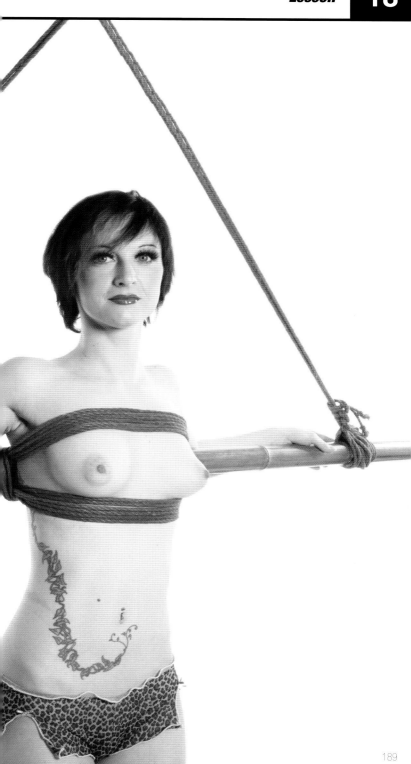

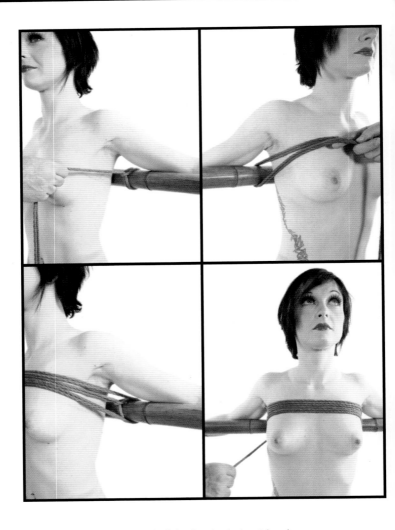

Position the bamboo behind the back at chest-level.

Start with a lark's head. then bring the rope across the upper chest.

Wrap the rope around the bamboo from the top and bring the rope back under the first wind.

Wrap the rope around the bamboo from the bottom and bring the rope across the upper chest (from the top) a final time.

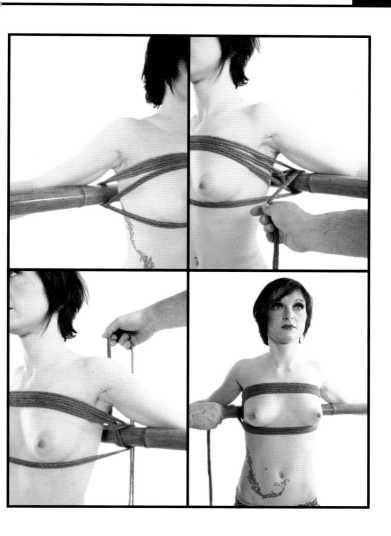

Wrap the rope around the bamboo from the top and bring it across under the breasts.

Wrap the rope around the bamboo from the bottom and anchor the upper ropes together.

Wrap the rope around the bamboo from the top in order to pass it a second time under the first rope beneath the breasts.

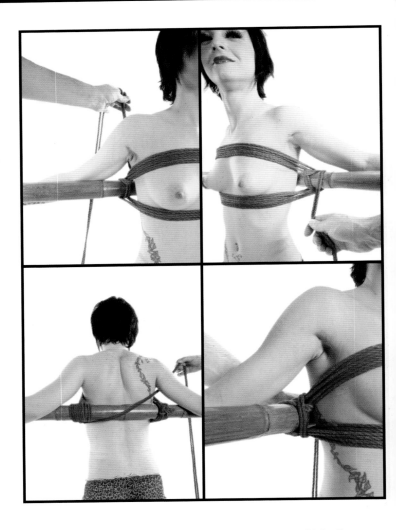

Wrap the rope around the bamboo from the bottom and take the upper ropes symmetrically to the other side.

Wrap the rope around the bamboo from the top and bring it a third time across the chest beneath the breasts.

Wrap the rope around the bamboo from the bottom and bring it up across the bamboo to the opposite side. Wrap the rope around the bamboo from the top.

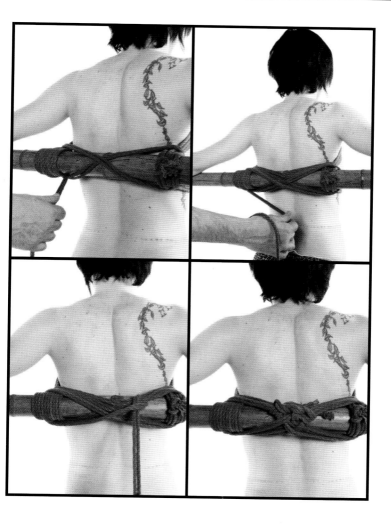

Continue forming figure-eights until you reach the rope's end, and finish with a series of overhand knots.

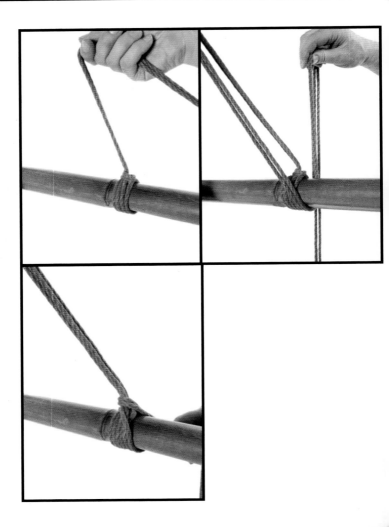

With a new rope and a lark's head, take the
bamboo just behind one of its nodes.
Wrap the rope once more, adjust the tension
then bring the rope up to the ring.

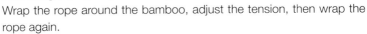

Wrap the rope around the bamboo, adjust the tension, then wrap the
rope again.

Finish with a series of overhand knots or wrap the rope a few more times
depending on the remaining length.

Attach the other side of the bamboo to the ring the same way.

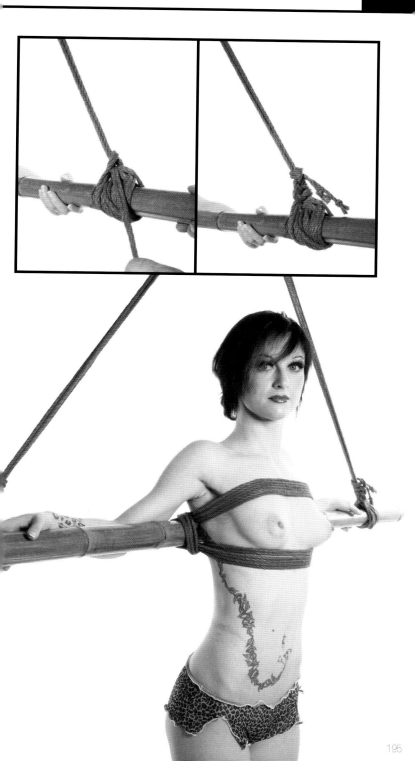

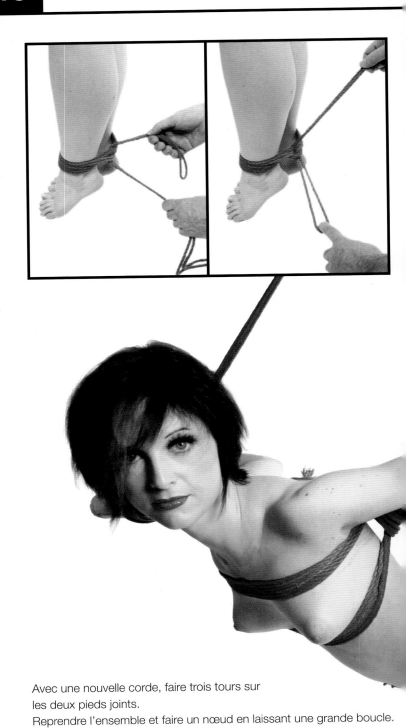

Avec une nouvelle corde, faire trois tours sur
les deux pieds joints.
Reprendre l'ensemble et faire un nœud en laissant une grande boucle.

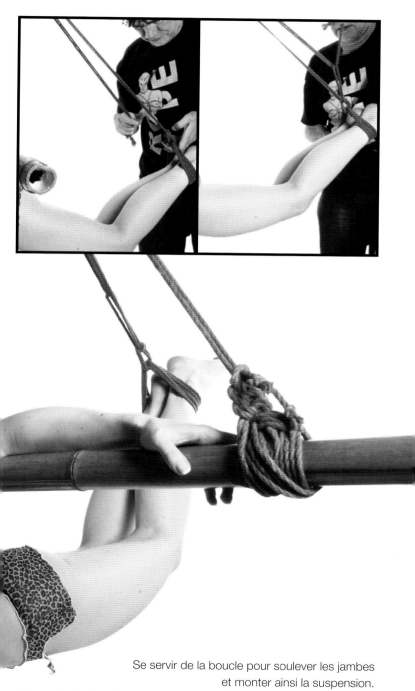

Se servir de la boucle pour soulever les jambes
et monter ainsi la suspension.
Reprendre la boucle et remonter pour bloquer au niveau de l'anneau.

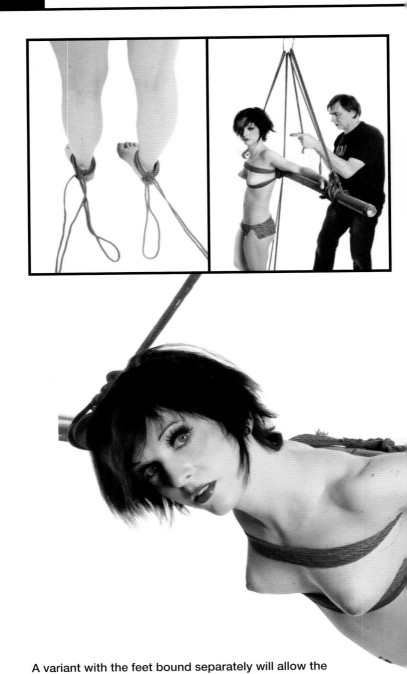

A variant with the feet bound separately will allow the
model further comfort and freedom of movement.

Wrap the rope three times around each ankle being sure to leave a
long bight.

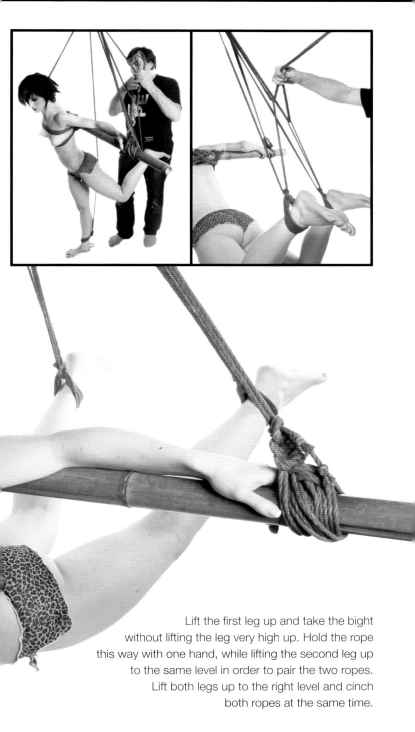

Lift the first leg up and take the bight without lifting the leg very high up. Hold the rope this way with one hand, while lifting the second leg up to the same level in order to pair the two ropes. Lift both legs up to the right level and cinch both ropes at the same time.

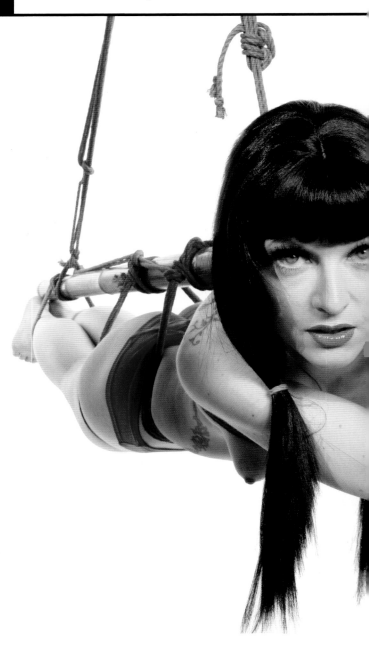

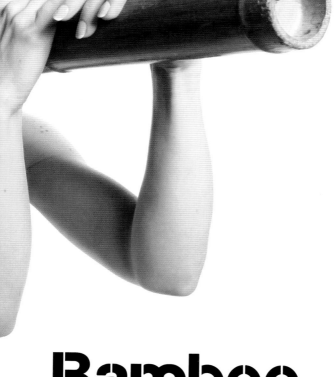

Bamboo
back
suspension

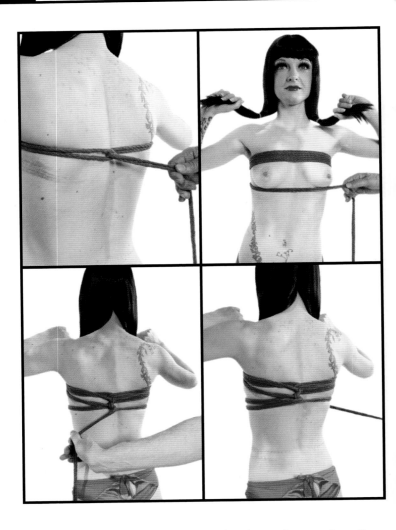

Start behind the back with a lark's head and wrap the rope three times above the breasts.

Repeat this below the breasts (three wraps).

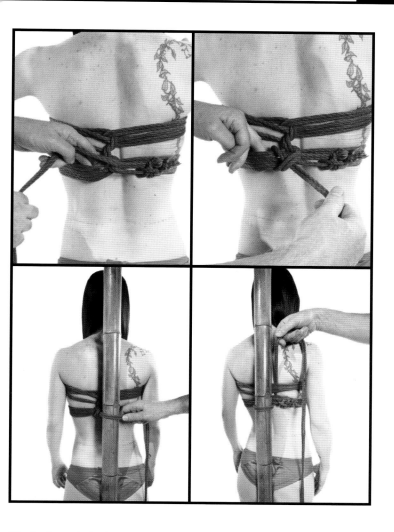

Cinch the whole lower wrap with an overhand knot. Position the bamboo behind the back.

Wrap the rope around the bamboo to affix it, and attach to all the back ropes.

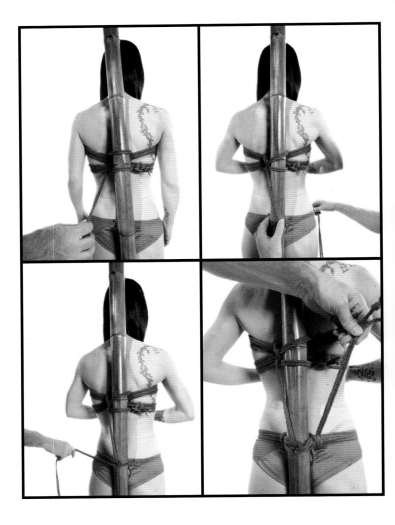

Wrap the rope once more around the bamboo and attach it to all the back ropes again.

Cinch here, then bring the rope down to the waist.

Wrap it around the waist twice and cinch the ropes onto the bamboo.

Leave this rope alone for the moment.

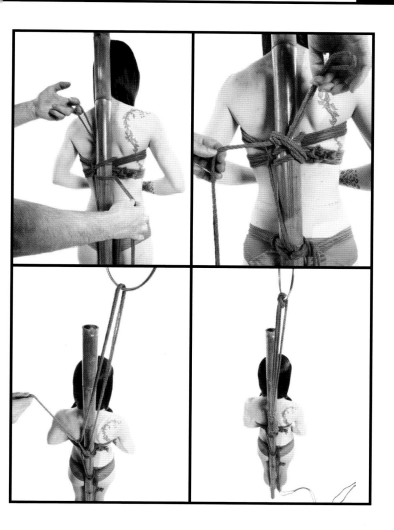

Before you continue around the legs, secure the model by linking this part to the suspension point.

Do this by wrapping a new rope behind the back in a figure eight that includes the bamboo and all ropes.

Tie a square knot as you leave a bight.

Run the rope through the ring and cinch.

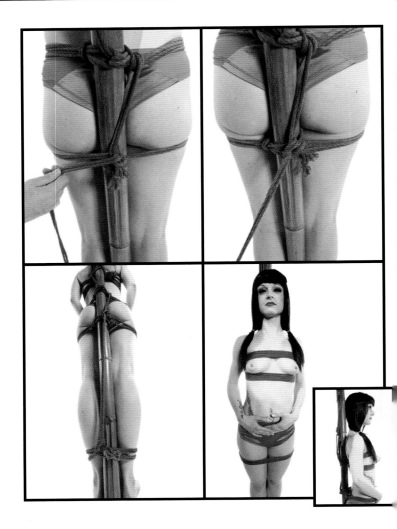

Continue around the legs with the rope that you left alone earlier.
Add another rope if needed.
Wrap the rope twice around the thighs, just under the buttocks.
Cinch it onto the bamboo and bring it down to the feet.
Wrap the rope twice around the ankles and cinch it to the bamboo.

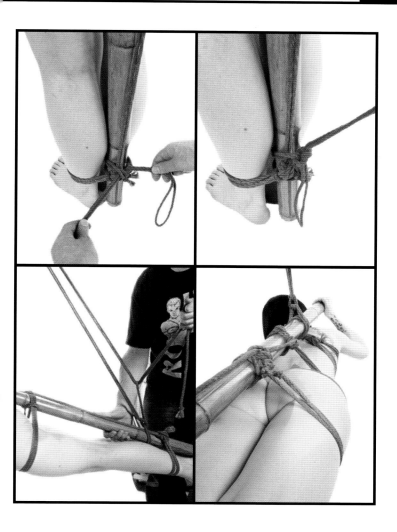

Wrap a new rope twice behind the bamboo to affix it as you leave a bight.

Lift the model up while holding the bamboo with one hand, take the bight then cinch onto the ring.

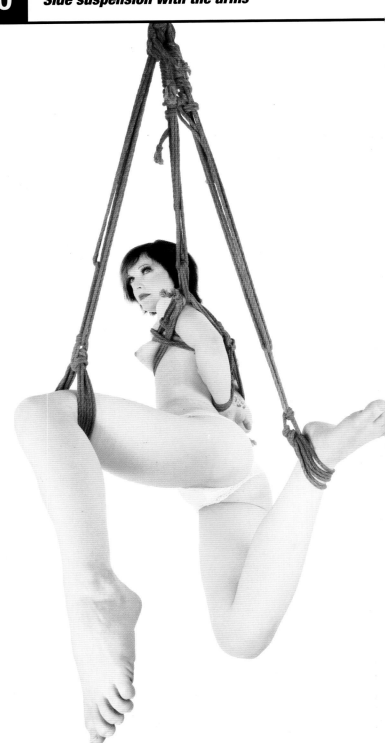

Side suspension with the arms

WARNING:

The next chapter demonstrates a side suspension that can be dangerous due to the position of the arms. This suspension risks damage to the nerves of the arm that bears the model's body weight. You must make sure the model doesn't experience any numbness, and you must only perform this suspension over a short length of time.

To relieve the model, you can untie the rope around the foot so she can use the floor for support.

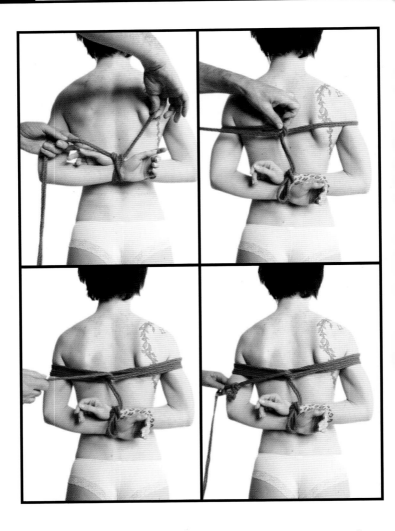

Start by wrapping the rope twice around the wrists, leaving a two-finger space between the wrists and ropes.

Next, wrap the rope three times above the breasts as you adjust the tension with each wind of the rope.

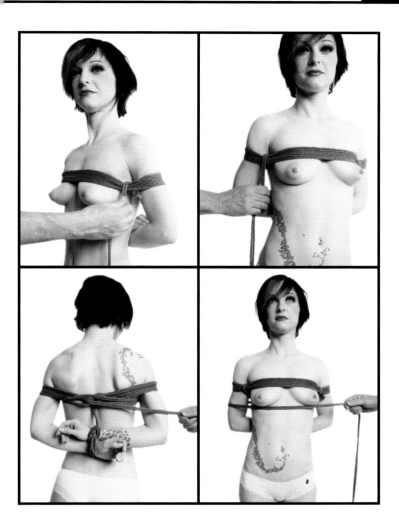

From top to bottom, pull the rope over the upper wrap between the chest and the arm.
Bring the rope across the back to the other side and do the same.
Adjust tension in the mid-back area, and bring the rope across the lower chest.

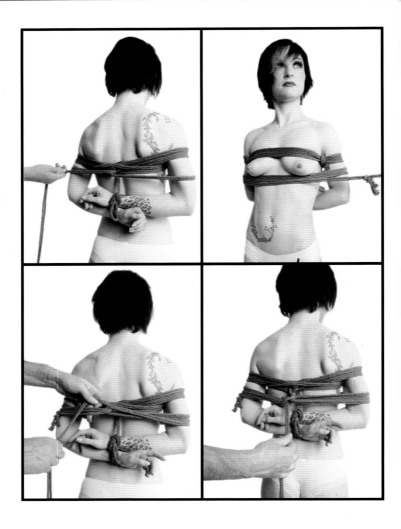

Wrap the rope three times below the breasts while using tension and counter-tension techniques, then cinch it mid-back.

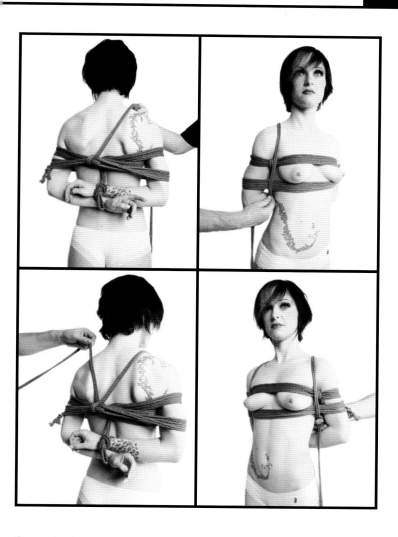

Create the first shoulder strap and bring the rope down straight between the chest and the arm to cinch the lower wrap. Adjust tension at the mid-back area, create the second shoulder strap, and repeat.

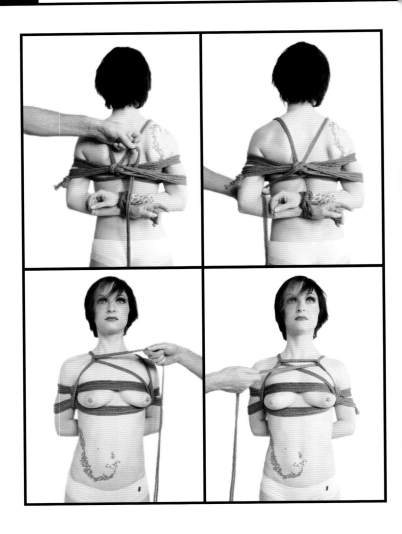

Tie an overhand knot.

Pull the rope through the space between the chest and the arm and include the opposite shoulder strap. Apply tension, then tuck the rope under the other shoulder strap in symmetry.

Bring the rope to the opposite side between the arm and the chest as you form a cross above the breasts.

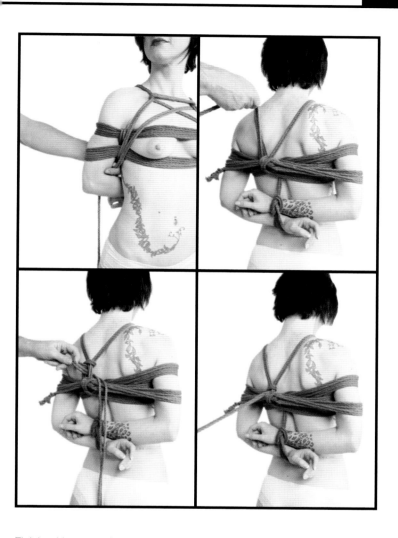

Finish with an overhand knot behind the back.

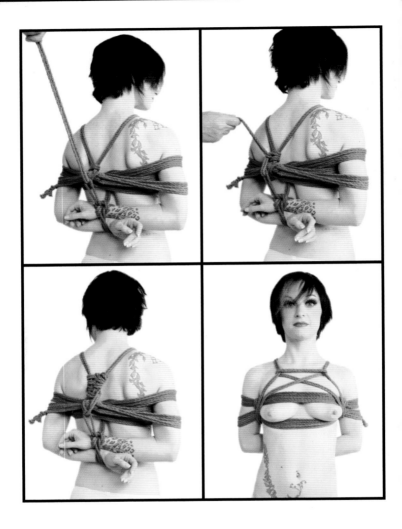

Take the bight that you had left on the wrists; cinch once again in mid-back and finish the rope aesthetically.

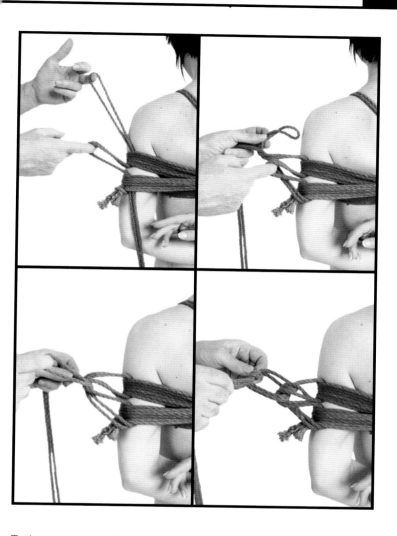

Tuck a new rope under the two wraps working from bottom to top, and leave a bight in between.

Connect all the ropes at the new bight and tie a square knot.

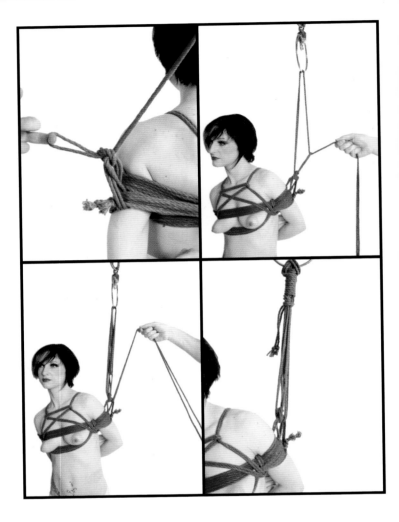

Bring the rope up to the suspension point then use the bight.
Bring the rope back up to the ring and pull it under the knot that holds the upper and lower wraps on the chest.
Return to the ring and cinch.

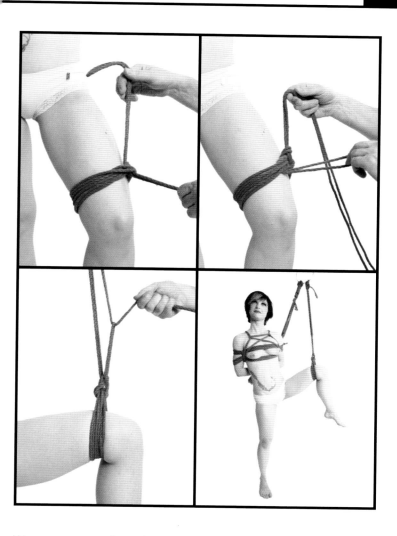

Wrap a new rope above the knee three times and tie a square knot.
Lift the leg up.
Run this rope through the ring, then bring it back down and use the bight.
Bring the rope back up to the ring and cinch.

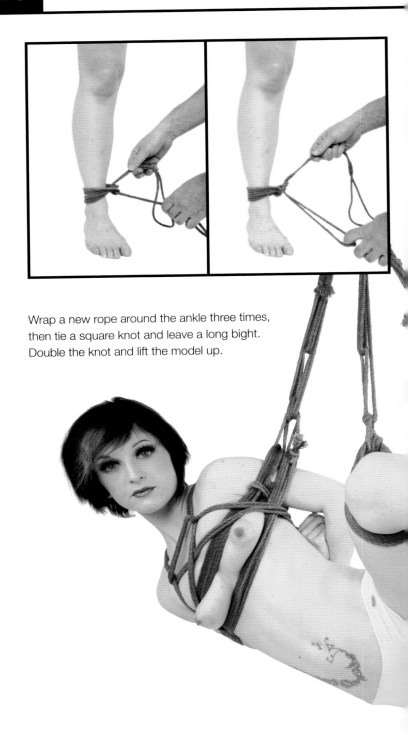

Wrap a new rope around the ankle three times,
then tie a square knot and leave a long bight.
Double the knot and lift the model up.

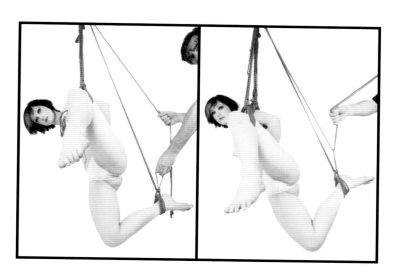

Use the bight and cinch the end of the rope onto the ring.

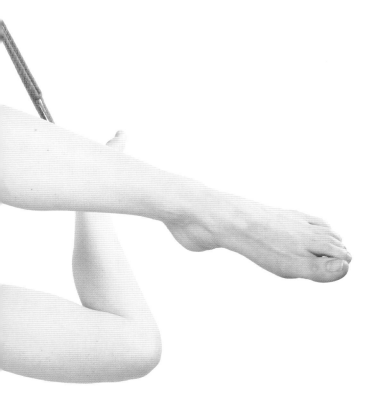

De Luxe Edition, panoramic format 28 cm x 24 cm on glossy paper, hard cover, English-French text, all the technique of Philippe Boxis plus a gallery of **100 art photographs presenting the author's performances.**

Please note: this edition contains full nude photos.

www.tabou-editions.com

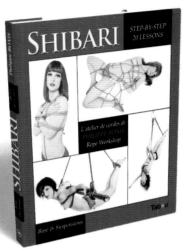

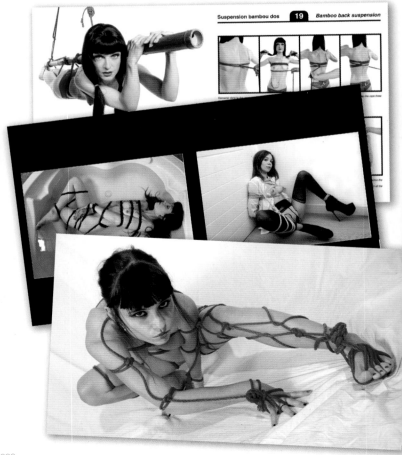

Acknowledgements

I would like to thank those who helped me to complete this book.

Thanks to Phoebus Kalista for the shots and to O. who worked as a model with kindness and availability for the whole technical part.

Thanks to Guy Berthier for my back cover photograph.

Thanks to David Ducarteron for his great work and to Xavier Duvet for his creativity and his friendship.

Thanks to the models who have, during these last ten years, shared this passion with me amongst closeness and happiness.

Thanks to Miia for her presence, her support and her help.

Thanks to Thierry Play of Tabou Editions for allowing this project to be realized.

Publisher
Tabou Éditions
91490 Milly-la-Forêt, France

Printer
Book Partners China Ltd
Chine